# Pocket Guide for the Home Care Aide

**Barbara Stover Gingerich, RN, MS, CHE, CHCE**
Consultant/Partner
ADVANTAGE Health Care Management Resources
Lititz, Pennsylvania

**Deborah Anne Ondeck, RN, MS, CPHQ, CHCE**
Consultant/Partner
ADVANTAGE Health Care Management Resources
Lititz, Pennsylvania

AN ASPEN PUBLICATION®
Aspen Publishers, Inc.
Gaithersburg, Maryland
1998

The authors have made every effort to ensure the accuracy of the information herein. However, appropriate information sources should be consulted, especially for new or unfamiliar procedures. It is the responsibility of every practitioner to evaluate the appropriateness of a particular opinion in the context of actual clinical situations and with due considerations to new developments. Authors, editors, and the publisher cannot be held responsible for any typographical or other errors found in this book.

**Library of Congress Cataloging-in-Publication Data**

Gingerich, Barbara Stover.
Pocket guide for the home care aide/Barbara Stover Gingerich,
Deborah Anne Ondeck.
p.    cm.
Includes bibliographical references and index.
ISBN 0-8342-1161-0
1. Home health aides—Handbooks, manuals, etc.    2. Nurses' aides—
Handbooks, manuals, etc.    I. Ondeck, Deborah Anne.    II. Title.
[DNLM: 1. Nurses' Aides handbooks.    2. Home Health Aides
handbooks.    WY 49G494p    1998]
RA645.3.G57    1998
362.1'4—dc21
DNLM/DLC
for Library of Congress
98-26061
CIP

Orders: (800) 638-8437
Customer Service: (800) 234-1660

**About Aspen Publishers** • For more than 35 years, Aspen has been a leading professional publisher in a variety of disciplines. Aspen's vast information resources are available in both print and electronic formats. We are committed to providing the highest quality information available in the most appropriate format for our customers. Visit Aspen's Internet site for more information resources, directories, articles, and a searchable version of Aspen's full catalog, including the most recent publications:
**http://www.aspenpublishers.com**
**Aspen Publishers, Inc.** • The hallmark of quality in publishing
Member of the worldwide Wolters Kluwer group.

Editorial Services: Joan Sesma
Library of Congress Catalog Card Number: 98-26061
ISBN: 0-8342-1161-0

*Printed in the United States of America*

1   2   3   4   5

This pocket guide is dedicated to the
thousands of paraprofessionals in recognition of
their unending gift of love, commitment, and caring
provided to the millions of individuals receiving
supportive health care in their homes.

# Table of Contents

# Preface

As a nurse aide working in the home health or hospice field, you encounter new people and situations every day. This pocket guide is lightweight and easy to carry with you in your car or in your bag. It contains important topics for you as you pursue your career in caring for patients in their home environment.

Working in the health care field means that you must understand:

- people and their differences
- yourself and how others see you
- growth and development for patients of all ages
- disease processes
- home care in general—the services, the payers, the family caregivers, and finally,
- procedures for giving safe care to your patients.

The *Pocket Guide for the Home Care Aide* contains topics of personal interest that you may want to sit and read when you have some time (for example, getting through an interview, identifying differences in people, learning to work well with people of all types, and the pros and cons of your work as a home care aide). When you are not reading it for pleasure, you will want to keep it close at hand to refer to while caring for your patients. The guide explains patient diagnoses and tells you what you should be watching for pertinent to a particular problem. Terms and definitions commonly used in home care are also provided. If you have a care plan with odd words on it, you can reference your pocket guide for assistance. This pocket guide does not replace your supervisor but rather brings information to you from others who have worked with home care aides.

You will notice that some sections contain blank lines for you to write what your agency does or how your supervisor wants you to handle a specific situation. Be sure to talk with your supervisor about these sections as you want to do what your employer requests. You can start to individualize this guide now:

My name is _____ .

If this book is lost, please call_____ .

We hope that you find this pocket guide to be a useful work tool. Enjoy reading and thank you for making a difference in the lives of home care patients.

# CHAPTER 1

# Orientation to Home Care

## THE HISTORY OF HOME CARE

As a home care aide, you are a special part of the health care provided to people in their homes. Think about the people you know who may be in need of help in their home. Some have signs of aging while others may be young but have ongoing health problems or a one-time serious illness. All of these people have one thing in common, though: They want to be able to live in their own home.

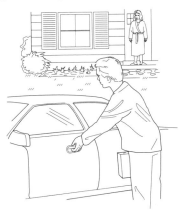

Health care has changed. In the early 1980s, people went to the hospital and stayed for several weeks. People had their operations and started to recover in the hospital. Now, for the same operation, they are in the hospital for only three or four days and are sent home (or somewhere else) to recover. Some of these patients need help with the tasks that other people do without thinking, such as preparing meals, eating, bathing, and dressing. This is where the home care aide helps. Home care aides are sent into homes to assist people with the physical care and home upkeep that they cannot do by themselves.

Home care is not new. It actually began in the 1700s in Boston. Women from a religious sect began to visit and care for sick people in their homes. This group, known as the Boston Dispensary, believed that sick people should not have to be sick and also sent away from the comfort of their home and family. It makes sense. Why should sick people have to give up the home and family that make them comfortable just because they need some help with personal care?

The roots of home care agencies, as we now know them, come from the VNAs (Visiting Nurse Associations) started in the late 1800s. The first opened in New York, and soon after others opened in major cities like Philadelphia and Boston. Before long, visiting nurse care also spread to the countryside. If you ever have a chance to visit a VNA, you will probably see pictures from its early years. There may be pictures of horse-drawn buggies with nurses wearing very starched uniforms. Imagine what it might have been like! Some had to walk miles and miles of mountain trails with a large "suitcase" full of supplies needed to help their patients. When they got to the home, they would have to pump water from the well—if they were lucky—or go down to the creek to bring up buckets of water to help bathe the patient. In those days, there were no home care aides. The nurses gave all of the care.

Today, there are many home care agencies in most larger communities. Some rural areas do not have home health care, which is a problem for people living there. Home care nurses still visit patients, but they do not help the patient with personal care activities of daily living anymore. Instead, the home care aide helps the patient with these activities.

## THE HISTORY OF HOSPICE

Dame Cicely Saunders developed the first hospice in England. During the early stages, patients with terminal diseases were sent to hospice buildings for care during their dying process. In the past 20 years, the hospice concept has spread to the United States. Instead of going to hospice buildings, though, the patients are cared for at home with the health care workers visiting them to provide care. Recently, hospice programs have started to have inpatient facilities, similar to the original hospices in England, and patients who do not have a 24-hour/day caregiver now have the option of hospice care in a safe environment.

## EMPLOYMENT OPPORTUNITIES FOR HOME CARE AIDES

There are a lot of opportunities for jobs in home care. In 1995, 18,874 home care agencies, including hospices, operated in the United States. All of them provide aide care to patients in their home. About 8,000 of them have aide positions in which the aide lives with a patient for a block of time. This is called private duty care or long-term care. In total, these agencies hire 215,220 home care aides (National Association for Home Care, 1997) at a salary range between $5.39 and $8.67 (National Association for Home Care, 1997).

In 1997, President Clinton saw that home care was growing very fast and became concerned that it was costing too much money. Based on spending, he thought that some home care providers were billing for care they never gave, so he put a four-month hold on approving new agencies for Medicare certification. Within the first month after the hold was lifted, 323 home care agencies applied for Medicare certification under tighter rules aimed at preventing fraud and abuse of the system.

As more Americans age, it is thought that home health care will continue to grow, and the care provided by the home care aide will be very important. Home care agencies are always looking for the right people to work as home care aides, for although many people can learn the skills needed, not everyone is right for a job as a home care aide. Home care aides must have energy and a pleasant personality. They should be able to learn the skills needed to care for patients living at home. Aides are guided by a nurse and need to follow the directions of the nurse. A good sense of humor and a compassionate personality help the aide to work with the elderly and sick. Looking ahead at what is needed and doing it without being asked makes patients and families happy. Good aides are those who want to help people, not just to earn a paycheck.

Home health agencies look for the following traits when hiring a home care aide:

- has good personality traits (e.g., caring, compassionate, pleasant, mature)
- wears clean clothing in good repair
- is clean and well-kept (personal hygiene)
- wears limited jewelry and make up
- is motivated to help people
- has a high energy level
- has dependable transportation (although staff may use public transportation or walk to their visits in some large cities)

- is able to read, write, and follow directions
- is willing to tell the nurse about the patient's condition
- has a sympathetic attitude toward the care of the sick

The fact that you have been hired by an agency means that you have or are expected to develop these qualities.

## ROLES IN HOME CARE AND HOSPICE SERVICES

Millions of patients are helped each year by a variety of health care workers in both home health care and hospice. Much of the care being provided to patients is by workers in your role. Your job is very important to home care and hospice patients.

### Home Care Roles

There are two levels of home health care services. The first level is professional services, also called skilled services, which are provided by someone with education after high school from specialty schools or colleges. Skilled services include

- physical therapy
- occupational therapy
- speech therapy

- social services
- nursing
- dietitians

The other level of care is called paraprofessional care or care that assists the skilled services. Titles for these jobs include

- home care aide
- certified nurses' aide
- homemaker/companion/live-in

To help you understand all of these roles, the following descriptions summarize what each one does.

### Physical Therapy

*Physical Therapists.* Physical therapy works with the bigger movements of the arms and legs. This therapy helps patients gain back their movements such as walking, getting out of bed, and bending stiff and sore joints. Physical therapists (PTs) ask patients to describe their problems and to give a history that explains why the problem exists. Questions asked might include the following:

- Did the patient have an operation?
- How long has the patient had this problem?
- When was the last time the patient was able to do the activity that he or she no longer can perform? What makes the joint hurt?

- What is the patient not able to do that he or she wants to do?

PTs also talk to the patient's physician about the patient's condition. After talking with the patient and physician, they plan some exercises that will help and teach them to the patient or do the exercises with the patient. Exercises make patients' muscles stronger and help them to be able to do the things they want to do. PTs often teach patients how to use mobility aids, such as wheelchairs, walkers, crutches, and canes. In the past physical therapists went to college. Now after college they must pass a written exam to be licensed to provide this type of skilled care.

*Physical Therapy Assistants.* Not all states permit physical therapy assistants (PTAs) to work in home health care. Some require that the PTA be directly supervised by a physical therapist on-site, which means that every time the PTA works with a patient the PT must be there. In home health care, this is not possible because the home care agency would need to pay both the PT and the PTA to make a visit, yet the agency can bill for only one visit. Physical therapy assistants are specially trained to help the therapist with modalities (heat packs, ice massage, ultrasound) and exercises. They work under the direction of the physical therapist, who also makes in-home supervisory visits to make sure that the PTAs are doing what needs to be done for the patient. PTAs do not develop the plan for care, nor do they assess the patient initially. PTAs go to college and pass an exam for licensure.

### Occupational Therapy

*Occupational Therapists.* The occupational therapist (OT) helps the patient to do everyday tasks known as activities of daily living. Activities of daily living include bathing, toileting, dressing, undressing, preparing meals, and doing light housework. Occupational therapists suggest the use of helping tools, called personal care aids, such as the following:

- *Sock aid.* The patient puts a sock over this sturdy yet bendable plate that has two straps attached to each side. The patient places a foot at the bendable plate and pulls the sock on with the help of the cloth straps.
- *Tub bench.* This bench has a plastic seat and rubber feet. When it is placed in the tub, the patient can sit while bathing. This helps patients to be safe when in the shower.
- *Extended shoe horn.* This shoe horn is approximately 12 inches long, and the patient uses it so that he or she does not have to bend to put shoes on.
- *Special utensils.* These knives, forks, and spoons are made with thick hand grips. Some are curved to help patients who cannot move their hands and arms well.

Occupational therapists go to college for four years, and in most states they must pass an exam for licensing.

*Certified Occupational Therapy Assistants.* Certified occupational therapy assistants (COTAs) take direction from occupational therapists, as PTAs do from PTs. Some state laws do not permit the use of COTAs, and those that do require that the OT make supervisory visits with COTAs and oversee what they do. COTAs perform exercises and training for activities of daily living. They go to college and then pass an exam for certification.

### Speech Therapy

The speech therapist (ST) is sometimes called a speech-language pathologist (SLP). This individual helps patients to relearn how to talk, read, write, and swallow. Speech therapy is helpful for patients with brain or nerve problems, such as a stroke or Parkinson's disease. Speech therapists must go to college for four years and work with an experienced therapist for one year after graduation to meet the Medicare requirements. They also pass an exam for licensing.

### Medical Social Services

The social worker helps patients with day-to-day problems that impact their health status. For example, when patients argue with their families or do not have money to buy food or anyone to take them to the physician, the social worker can help by talking with them. Social workers know about helpful agencies in the community and can make referrals to agencies equipped to provide food, money, medications, or transportation to physician offices. Social workers help patients who are not able to do the things they used to be able to do. Sometimes just talking with specially trained people who are outside of their family can be just what the patient needs. To become a social worker, four or five years of college are needed. Many states also require the social worker to pass an exam for licensing.

### Nursing

Registered nurses (RNs) provide most of the professional home care visits to patients. The services provided by the RN include

- teaching patients and their families or caregivers
- evaluating patient conditions
- doing procedures, such as wound care or drawing blood for lab work
- overseeing the care of a patient with many illnesses

RNs go to school for two to five years. After completing their schooling, nurses must pass a state exam to be licensed to provide nursing care.

LPNs/LVNs (licensed practical nurses/licensed vocational nurses) work with RNs in home care. These nurses usually go to school for one year. They do some of the same things that the RN does, such as checking blood pressures, doing wound care, and teaching patients. The LPN/LVN does not admit patients into the home care agency or provide complicated care.

### Dietitians

The role of the dietitian has taken on more importance over the past several years. Dietitians either assist the patient directly or work with the nurse, who then assists the patient. They specialize in nutrition. Dietitians evaluate the intake of the patient; educate nurses, patients, and caregivers regarding special diets; and assist in the evaluation of the nutritional care plan. Dietitians go to college for four years and pass an exam for licensure.

### Home Care Aide

This person helps with the patient's hygiene needs and provides some light house cleaning. This is the role you fill as part of the home care team. The title home care aide (HCA) was adopted by the National Association for Home Care (NAHC), which is a group whose members are home care agencies. Home care aides are trained to do specific tasks, need to pass an exam, and are observed providing personal care tasks. Once aides pass the test, they are certified or approved to care for Medicare and Medicaid patients. This will be discussed in more detail later.

### Certified Nurses' Aide

Some states want all aides in the state to take the same test. In these states the state, rather than the agency, prepares the test questions and scores the tests. These states then give aides a certificate and wallet card showing that they are certified or approved in that state. This test also covers the topics that Medicare and Medicaid require.

### Homemaker/Companion/Live-In Companion

Different agencies use these different titles for other jobs in home care. Usually, these individuals do not help the patient with bathing but do more in the area of cleaning and preparing meals. In some agencies, the person remains with the patient in case the patient falls or needs help.

## Hospice Roles

### Medical Director

The medical director works closely with the hospice team. This physician also assists other physicians by educating them about the purpose of hospice and providing them with the newest information on how to control pain, one of the major goals of hospice care. The medical director attends team meetings and in some agencies has a more active role, such as visiting patients and directing all of their care. In some cases, home care agencies also have a medical director.

### Bereavement Coordinator/Counselor

This individual helps the family and caregiver(s) cope with the patient's death. In most agencies this person did not work directly with the patient, and therefore the family shares more. This person never knew the deceased patient but is very interested in learning about him or her.

### Spiritual Counselor

The spiritual counselor may be a hired member of the team, such as a priest, minister, or rabbi, or the patient's personal clergyperson. A hospice must have someone available to address patients' spiritual needs at this point in their lives if the patient and/or family desires.

### Social Worker

Social workers help the patient to cope with terminal illness. They visit hospice patients more often than they visit home care patients. They use their education to decide when and how to discuss patients' conditions with them and what to include in the discussion. The social worker is not the only member of the hospice team assisting the patient with coping. Actually, every member of the hospice team is specially trained to address the situation.

## WHO PAYS THE BILL?

Health maintenance organizations (HMOs) pay for limited home health care services for their clients, and every year, more people sign up for health care coverage from HMOs. HMOs have someone who acts as a gate-keeper, called a case manager. The case manager's job is to talk with the home care agency staff to find out about the patient. Based on this information, the case manager tells the agency the number of visits for which the HMO will pay. Agencies are sometimes upset because they think that the patient needs more visits than what the case manager approves. For this reason, the government passed a law saying that HMOs must pay for home health care services, especially in certain situations. For example, if new mothers go home from the hospital within 48 hours from when they have the baby, they must be offered one home nursing visit. Usually, HMOs do not pay for home care aides because they do not pay for bathing, cooking, and similar services.

## Home Health Care Payers

### *Insurance*

Most insurance companies pay for home health care services, including aide care. Few traditional policies pay for private duty or long-term care. Some companies have long-term care policies that pay for home health care for people with sickness that gets worse over time. This type of home care is called long-term care or private duty. Usually, aides or nurses stay with the patient for blocks of time, such as four hours, eight hours, or longer.

### Medicaid (Medical Assistance)

Medical assistance (MA) provides health care for the poor. The money comes from the government. Each state plans what MA will cover and what it will not cover. The federal government requires that states pay for nursing and aide care. Other services are up to the state. For that reason, what one state pays for, other states may not cover. Most states cover home care aides. Since there are many poor people who depend on MA for health care and since the states only have a small amount of money for MA, many states limit the number of visits for which they will pay for each patient during a month.

MA also pays for special services for certain illnesses under MA waiver services. For example, people with AIDS (acquired immune deficiency syndrome) who are covered by MA in Pennsylvania can get many kinds of services that would not be covered by MA alone. They also have a case manager. This case manager is hired by MA to talk with patients and evaluate them. If an AIDS patient is losing a lot of weight, MA waiver services include meal supplements. Also, AIDS patients can have skilled services (nursing and therapy) and long-term home care aide services (up to eight hours at a time, if needed). Other waiver services vary from state to state.

### *Medicare*

Medicare covers home health care for people over 65 and younger people with long-term disabilities. For Medicare to pay for home care services:

- The patient needs to be confined to the home because of a mental or physical condition. The illness must be current. For example, some people have heart trouble for years. Medicare will pay for home care only if the heart trouble is acute (severe but not recurrent or lasting a long time). For instance, if the patient's blood pressure goes up or if the patient has chest pain that he or she did not have before, the illness is acute.
- The patient must need care that Medicare considers to be skilled care; that is, the patient must need the services of a nurse or therapist. If the patient needs those services, then Medicare will pay for aides and social workers if the patient has a need for them as well.
- The patient must not need care for more than 8 hours per day or 28 hours per week.

In the *Health Insurance Manual for Home Health Care* (HIM 11) (HCFA, 1995), it is clear that Medicare pays for the home care aide to give primarily personal care and other care in conjunction with personal care. Medicare includes the following in home care aide services:

1. personal care, including the following services that are provided to facilitate treatment or prevent deterioration:
   - bathing
   - dressing
   - grooming
   - caring for hair
   - nail care
   - oral hygiene for the patient's health
   - changing the bed linens of an incontinent patient
   - shaving
   - deodorant application
   - skin care with lotions and/or powder
   - foot care
   - ear care
   - feeding
   - assistance with elimination (including enemas unless the skills of a licensed nurse are required due to the patient's condition)
   - routine catheter care
   - routine colostomy care
   - assistance with ambulation
   - changing position in bed
   - assistance with transfers

2.  simple dressing changes that do not require the skills of a licensed nurse

3.  assistance with medications that are ordinarily self-administered and do not require the skills of a licensed nurse to be provided safely and effectively

4.  assistance with activities that are directly supportive of skilled therapy services but do not require the skills of a therapist to be safely and effectively performed, such as
    *   routine maintenance exercises
    *   repetitive practice of functional communication skills to support speech-language pathology services

5.  routine care of prosthetic and orthotic devices

Under Medicare, when a home care aide visits a patient to provide a health-related service, as listed above, the home care aide may also perform some incidental services that do not meet the definition of a home care aide service (e.g., light cleaning, preparation of a meal, taking out the trash, shopping). However, the purpose of a home care aide visit may not be to provide these incidental services, since they are not health-related services but rather are necessary household tasks that must be performed by anyone to maintain a home.

Medicare is changing the way it pays home care agencies. It used to pay agencies what it cost to care for each patient. Now Medicare pays a preset amount for each patient visit. It is important to understand this, because it explains why home care agencies need to change the way they operate. To make this change easier to understand, pretend that you own a grocery store. The Jones family buys groceries from you every week, and they pay for each grocery item they buy. Let's say that every week, the Joneses paid an average of $75 two years ago, $85 last year, and $100 this year. As the grocery store owner, if you were paid the way Medicare is paying home care agencies, you would now be paid only $90 a week. If the Jones family had company coming and they needed more groceries one week, you would still get $90. As a grocery store owner, you hope that another family will need fewer groceries than it usually does to help you make up the extra that the Jones family needs. In home care you may be asked if you think that any of your patients can be cared for with fewer visits. Your agency needs to make sure that they save some money somewhere to provide more visits to patients with more needs.

### Self-Pay

As people age and become dependent on care that is not paid for by insurance, they sometimes pay for the care out of their own pocket. To stay at home, more people are using their savings to pay for health care. Usually they chose to spend their money on care provided by home care aides, homemakers, companions, and live-in helpers.

### *Other*

There are other sources that pay for home health care. Other types of payers include PPOs (preferred provider organizations) and PHOs (physician-hospital organizations). Other government funding is also available for paraprofessional services (home care aide, etc.), and some community organizations, like the MS Society, sometimes pay for services as well. Home care agencies are always looking for new sources of payment for their services.

## Hospice Payers

Hospice services include medical, nursing, aide, counseling, bereavement, and (if needed) dietary and therapy services. The goal of these services is comfort. People who have had all of the treatment that they want or that is available for their condition have the option of selecting hospice care. To make sure that patient rights are maintained, hospice explains the purpose of its services and asks patients to sign a form showing that they were educated about the difference between home care and hospice.

Hospice services are paid for by the same payers as home care. Most payers require that the patient have a prognosis (life span) of 6 to 12 months or less. Three types of payers and some of their requirements for hospice follow:

1. *Medicare.*
   - Patients and family/caregiver are admitted to the program.
   - Medicare pays the hospice for every day of service in these areas:
     - routine—day-to-day care and services needed for the patient
     - continuous—predominantly nursing care delivered at times of crises to care for the medical needs of the patient
     - respite—care given in the absence of the family/caregivers to allow them time to relax
     - inpatient—short hospitalizations for pain control or other medical crises
   - The physician must sign a statement that the patient's prognosis is six months or less.
   - Medicare pays for medication related to the terminal condition.
   - It pays for medical equipment needed to care for the patient (e.g., hospital bed, bedside commode).
   - Care planning must be done by the entire team.

- Bereavement services must be available for a 12-month period for the family and caregivers after the patient dies.
2. *Medical assistance.* Medical assistance is controlled by the individual states, and its requirements are similar to those of Medicare.
3. *Insurance/HMOs/other.* These payers have various hospice packages, but generally the coverage is similar to Medicare.

## THE HOME CARE/HOSPICE TEAM

To run smoothly, home health agencies need all workers to get their jobs done on time. It is like a machine or assembly line where one job is dependent on the next, which is dependent on the next, and so forth. So who are the team members? The team includes the patient and every care provider:

- physician
- home care aides
- homemakers
- companions
- live-ins
- nurses
- therapists

- social workers
- dietitians
- caregiver/family

The team also includes office support services, such as

- intake staff
- schedulers
- supply clerks
- billers
- payroll clerks
- administrator

In addition to the above, the hospice team includes

- medical director
- bereavement coordinator/counselor
- spiritual counselor

After evaluating the patient's condition, the physician orders care for the patient by writing down and signing for the kind of care that the patient needs. The physician also is available to talk with the agency nurse or supervisor about the patient's condition.

The home care aide works most closely with the scheduler and one or two nurses. At times, the therapist might meet the home care aide in the home and teach the aide how to move the patient or help the patient exercise. It is important to remember that every job and every person is part of the team. Without each one of the workers, the patient would not receive high-quality care.

Home care aides play one of the most important roles in home care. They are the ones who spend the most time with the patients. They also help patients with the little things that mean so much and make their day. Think about how you would feel if you could not put on your shoes or make a meal. Patients are thankful that you do these things for them. Since you help patients with so many things, they often tell you things that they do not tell the nurse or the therapist. They might think that the nurse is too busy to talk with them or is not interested. They feel better talking with an aide because they feel more comfortable. This special relationship between the home care aide and the patient places a big responsibility on the aide, making the aide a central person in the home care team.

It is very important that you let the nurse know about problems that the patient tells you about. The information you provide to the nurse may become part of the patient's care plan.

## CARE PLANNING

The care plan lists

- all of the patient's problems related to his or her medical condition

- care that the home care team will provide to the patient
- goals of care

Figure 1–1 diagrams the care planning process.

Care planning is done differently in each agency. Some agencies and hospices have regular face-to-face team meetings to discuss the patient and his or her condition. In some agencies, team members call a selected team member, usually the registered nurse, and provide information about the patient's problems, planned interventions, and goals for care. Patient problems may be stated as

- medical diagnoses (e.g., myocardial infarction)
- nursing diagnoses (e.g., inability to ambulate secondary to fracture)
- problem list (e.g., insufficient income)

Problems you share with the team may need to be placed on the patient's care plan so that all team members are aware of the problem and each approaches the problem in a similar way. For example, Joe Smith is unable to buy his medicine toward the end of the month because he runs out of money. This problem is put on the care plan along with interventions by the social worker and the nurse. Table 1–1 is a sample team care plan for the patient in which the problems, care provided, and goals are all listed on one piece of paper.

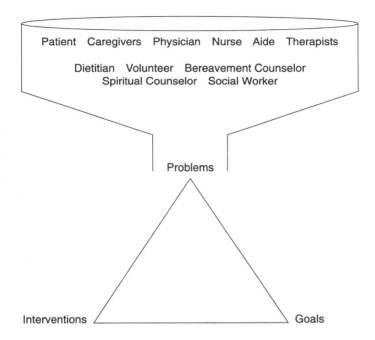

Patient Caregivers Physician Nurse Aide Therapists

Dietitian Volunteer Bereavement Counselor
Spiritual Counselor Social Worker

Problems

Interventions

Goals

**Figure 1–1** Care Planning Process. *Source:* Reprinted with permission from ADVANTAGE Health Care Management Resources.

In addition to the team care plan, the registered nurse prepares a very detailed aide care plan. Exhibit 1–1 is a sample aide care plan that shows the specific kinds of patient personal care the aide is to provide. For example, Mr. Smith is to have a bedbath. If Mr. Smith is feeling

**Table 1–1** Team Care Plan

Patient Name: <u>Joe Smith</u>

| Problem | Discipline | Care | Goals |
|---------|-----------|------|-------|
| Myocardial infarction | Nurse | Assess blood pressure and vital signs 3× per week × 2 weeks then 1–2× per week × 3 weeks. Instruct patient regarding new medications with each visit. Assess pain severity, frequency, and duration with each visit. | Stable cardiac condition (BP below 150/90 within 5 weeks, pulse regular and between 60 and 90 within 2 weeks, no episodes of chest pain within 5 weeks) |
| Weakness | Physical therapist | Develop a progressive home exercise program and educate patient during visits 1× per week × 3 weeks. Assess strength and range of motion with every visit. | Increased strength in bilateral quadriceps 4+ within 3 weeks |
| | | Give personal care 3× per week × 3 weeks then reevaluate need. | Maintenance of good personal hygiene |

continues

**Table 1–1** continued

Patient Name: Joe Smith

| Problem | Discipline | Care | Goals |
|---|---|---|---|
| Financial problems | Social worker | Educate patient regarding community resources to assist with medication purchases during 1 visit. | Purchase of medications for entire month |
| | Nurse | Assess medication use by counting medications with every visit. | Medications taken as prescribed on an ongoing basis |

*Source:* Reprinted with permission from ADVANTAGE Health Care Management Resources.

**Exhibit 1–1** Aide Care Plan

| Patient: Joe Smith | | | | Aide: Abbey Brown | SOC: 8/9/98 | Payer: MC | |

| Care | Frequency | Complete | Assist as needed | Care | Frequency | Complete | Assist as needed |
|---|---|---|---|---|---|---|---|
| Bed bath | Mon., Wed., Fri. (wk. 1) | | ✓ | Bedpan use | | | |
| Sink bath | Mon., Wed., Fri. (wk. 2) | | ✓ | Urinal use | | | |
| Tub bath/shower | Mon., Wed., Fri. (wk. 3) | | ✓ | Toileting, bathroom | Mon., Wed., Fri. for 3 wks. | | ✓ |
| Shave | Mon., Wed., Fri. for 3 wks. | | | Blood pressure | Mon., Wed., Fri. for 3 wks. | ✓ | |
| Shampoo bed/sink Shower | Mon., Wed., Fri. (wk. 3) | | ✓ | Vital signs | Mon., Wed., Fri. for 3 wks. | ✓ | |
| Nail care | | | | Meal preparation | | | |
| Skin care | | | | Cleaning | | | |
| Assist with dressing | Mon., Wed., Fri. for 3 wks. | | ✓ | Laundry | | | |
| Transfer assistance | Mon., Wed., Fri. for 3 wks. | | ✓ | Other | | | |
| Ambulation | | | | Other | | | |

**Exhibit 1–1** continued

**Explanation/Special Instructions:** Use only an electric razor. Report any bleeding to the nurse.

Report BP > 150/90. Report temperature > 101°F. Report pulse < 60 or > 90.

Report any complaints of chest pain or other problems.

**Medications:** Heart pill—daily. Water pill—twice a day. Blood pressure pill—daily.

Blood thinner—daily. Vitamin—daily

**Directions:** Turn right out of parking lot to route 66. Turn left on route 66 to exit 23 (route 47).

At the end of the ramp, turn left onto route 47. Travel exactly 2.2 miles to the big white farmhouse

just past the pond.

**Prepared by:** _Nancy Nurse, RN_    **Date:** _8/9/98_

really good and asks to be seated on the commode for a sink bath, the aide must call the nurse or supervisor for permission. The aide must not change the kind of care provided but must follow the instructions, which are often ordered by the physician.

# CHAPTER 2

# Definitions and Terminology

## COMMON HOME CARE TERMS

The following list of terms includes diets and terminology that you may see written on the patient's record. Your organization may have additional terminology that it uses frequently. Use the space at the end of this section to add terms to your pocket guide.

**Abuse**—Hurting someone or something. There are different kinds of abuse:

- verbal abuse: making fun of someone to hurt them; using foul language
- physical abuse: hitting or touching a person in a hurtful way
- sexual abuse: forcing someone to take part in sexual activity
- child abuse: hurting someone under the age of 18
- elder abuse: hurting someone in the older age group (e.g., 60 or older)

**Accreditation**—A process whereby an organization evaluates the way the agency does business and, if services follow the standards (rules) set by the organization, grants the agency approval.

**Activities of daily living**—The things that people must do every day to take care of their bodies. These include bathing, brushing teeth, combing hair, toileting, dressing, undressing, eating, and drinking.

**Acute**—This term is used with diagnoses. It means that the patient's condition just began or just became worse and the patient can get better with treatment. Some examples of acute diagnoses are heart attacks, gallstones, and bronchitis.

**ADA diet (American Diabetic Association Diet)**—This is a well-balanced diet and includes foods from all five food groups. No concentrated sugars are permitted (e.g., candy, pie).

**Caregiver**—Any person who gives care to the patient. This can be a family member, friend, or agency employee.

**Care plan**—The written directions listing the patient's problems, what the staff need to do for the patient, and goals for the care. The aide's care plan is written and changed only by the nurse.

**Case manager**—The individual responsible for directing the care received by the patient. Case managers work for payers, home care agencies, and community service organizations.

**Catheter**—A tube that is inserted into the patient to drain or insert fluids. (For example, a urinary catheter is put into the urinary bladder to drain urine; an angio-catheter is put into the vein for fluids and medicines to be instilled.)

**Certified nurses' aide**—A person with state approval to work in the state as a home care aide.

**Chronic**—This term is used with diagnoses. It means that the patient's condition is long term, maybe even life-long. Some examples of chronic diagnoses are arthritis, diabetes, and emphysema.

**Companion**—The person who stays with the patient. The duties of the companion vary from agency to agency but do not include personal care. Usually a companion stays with the patient in case there is a problem.

**Culture**—A group with similar beliefs, morals, and tra-ditions.

**Diagnosis**—This is another term for illnesses or disabilities. Some example of diagnoses are colds, diabetes, and cancer.

**Disability**—The person is unable to do what most people can do without difficulty. For example, the person may not be able to hear or walk.

**Documentation**—Writing down what happened at a point in time. Home care aides need to write down what they helped the patient with during the visit.

**Edema**—Excessive fluid collection in areas of the body. The aide needs to look for edema in patients' feet and ankles and, if found, report it to the nurse.

**Ethics**—Deals with and attempts to resolve moral problems.

**Ethnicity**—The combined characteristics of individuals having to do with the region and country from which they came.

**Health care worker**—Anyone who provides direct patient care (e.g., home care aide, nurse, therapist, social worker, etc.)

**Hemiplegic**—Not able to move one side of the body. This is usually caused by a stroke.

**HMO (health maintenance organization)**—These companies contract with people to pay for their health and medical care. HMOs pay for services to keep the patient in good health and not just to get them back to good health once they become sick.

**Homebound**—Unable to leave the home because of a medical or psychiatric illness. If the homebound patient does leave the home, it should be rarely and it takes a lot of effort. Homebound status is used by Medicare and Medicaid in some states to determine whether to pay for home care services.

**Home care aide**—The person who is trained to meet Medicare/Medicaid standards to help patients with their personal care needs.

**Homemaker**—The person who helps the patient with meal preparation, cleaning, and laundry. Other duties of this position vary from agency to agency.

**Hospice**—Care given to patients with serious and terminal illness. Payers have different rules about who qualifies for hospice care. The rules usually say that the patient should have a prognosis of 6–12 months, or less, for hospice to be covered.

**Instrumental activities of daily living**—The things that people need to do to be independent, including preparing meals, using the telephone, cleaning, doing laundry, shopping, and making change.

**Live-in helper**—The person who stays with the patient around the clock. The duties of this position vary from agency to agency. Usually, the live-in helper is responsible for keeping the home in order and preparing meals for the patient.

**NAS diet (no added salt diet)**—Patients with heart, liver, and kidney problems are placed on a NAS diet. Patients on a NAS diet should not eat salty foods such as potato chips, pickles, and processed cheeses. They should not add salt at the table and should use very small amounts in cooking.

**Neglect**—Not helping or doing things that need to be done for a person or animal. Neglect can be emotional or physical.

**Order**—This is the action that one person directs another to do. For example, physicians order nurses to evaluate patients and therapists to teach patients how to increase their strength.

**Organic brain syndrome**—This is another term for senility and is caused by brain cells being damaged by aging.

**Outcome**—Result of an action. In home care, one outcome to the home care aide visit is a clean patient.

**Paralyzed**—Not able to move a part or parts of the body.

**Paraplegic**—Not able to move the lower extremities.

**Payer**—The person or company paying for services and care. In health care, payers are usually insurance companies, Medicare, Medicaid, HMOs, and individuals.

**Personality trait**—A characteristic of a person's behavior, for example, assertive, aggressive, or passive.

**Phlebotomy** (fla-bot-a-me)—Putting a needle into a vein to draw blood samples.

**Prognosis**—The feasibility of recovery, as in good or poor; the time that the physician thinks the patient has left to live (stated in days, weeks, months, or years).

**Quadraplegic**—Unable to move all four extremities (arms and legs).

**Supervisory visit**—This is a visit made to the home to determine the patient's opinion about the care and/or observe a home care worker giving care. Medicare requires that supervisory visits be made for home care aide services.

**2 gm. sodium (Na) diet**—Patients with severe heart, liver, or kidney disease are asked to limit their sodium (salt) intake to 2000 mg. The patient should read the ingredients listed on labels and add up the amount of sodium in the foods he or she is eating. The dietitian can give the patient a list of foods and sodium amounts for planning.

**Universal precautions**—National rules set by the Centers for Disease Control and Prevention to prevent the spread of infection. Some examples of the rules are the need to wear gloves, aprons, and so forth when giving patients certain types of care.

**Venipuncture**—Putting a needle into a vein to draw blood for testing. This is also called phlebotomy.

Other terms from your organization:

_____

_____

_____

_____

_____

## DIAGNOSES

The following is a partial list of some of the diagnoses you might see on the patient's record:

**A-Fib**—Atrial fibrillation. A bad rhythm in the heart. The smaller chambers (the atria), beat very fast. Patients can develop blood clots from this bad rhythm.

**AIDS**—Acquired immune deficiency syndrome. A blood disorder without a cure.

**AKA**—Above knee amputation. The removal of the foot, lower leg, and knee. Often performed as a result of poor circulation or trauma.

**ALL**—Acute lymphocytic leukemia. A blood disorder where white blood cells die before they mature enough to fight infection. This disease often ends in death unless it goes into remission (corrects itself for a period of time).

**ASCAD**—Arteriosclerotic coronary artery disease. Hardening of the arteries in the heart.

**ASCVD**—Arteriosclerotic cardiovascular disease. Hardening of the arteries in the body.

**ASHD**—Arteriosclerotic heart disease. Hardening of the arteries in the heart.

**ASMI**—Anterioseptal myocardial infarction. A heart attack in the front portion of the heart (largest portion) and the tissue that separates the sides of the heart.

**AVR**—Aortic valve replacement. An artificial valve replacement between the left atrium and left ventricle.

**AWMI**—Anterior wall myocardial infarction. A heart attack in the front portion of the heart (largest portion).

**BBB**—Bundle branch block. An irregular heart beat resulting from the ventricle not getting an electrical message sent by the atria.

**BKA**—Below knee amputation. Surgical removal of the foot and lower leg. The knee is not removed, which makes walking with an artificial leg easier.

**BPD**—Broncho-pulmonary dysplasia. A lung disease caused by premature birth. It usually goes away by age two or three.

**BPH**—Benign prostatic hypertrophy. An inflammation of the prostate caused by something other than cancer.

**BSO**—Bilateral salpingo oophorectomy. The surgical removal of a woman's ovaries and fallopian tubes.

**Bx.**—Biopsy. A sample of the tissue or cells that is removed from the patient and sent to the lab for diagnostic analysis under a microscope.

**CA**—Cancer. A disease in which abnormal cells grow very rapidly and take over for functioning cells.

**CABG**—Coronary artery bypass graft. A transplanted artery from one area (usually the leg) into the heart to permit circulation in an area with a clogged artery.

**CAD**—Coronary artery disease. Disease of the arteries in the heart (usually as a result of blockage).

**CAI**—Coronary artery ischemia. A poor blood supply to the heart.

**CLL**—Chronic lymphocytic leukemia. A blood disorder effecting the white cells. The patient has chronic vague symptoms, such as fatigue, swollen glands, lack of appetite, fever, and enlarged liver and spleen. Patients can live a long time with this type of leukemia. It is usually found in people between the ages of 50 and 70.

**CML**—Chronic myelogenous leukemia. A blood disorder caused by faulty bone marrow formation of white blood cells. Symptoms include enlarged liver and spleen, pain in the long bones, and weight loss with weakness. Usually found in people ages 20–40.

**CMV**—Cytomegalovirus. A virus that attacks the eyes. It is seen often in AIDS patients.

**COPD**—Chronic obstructive pulmonary disease. Also known as emphysema, this is a disease of the lungs in which the air sacs lose their elasticity, resulting in shortness of breath, wheezing, and a productive cough.

**Cor. Insuff.**—Coronary insufficiency. Poor blood supply to the heart muscle.

**CP**—Cerebral palsy. A disease or injury to the nerve tissue in the brain that causes muscle paralysis.

**CPR**—Cardiopulmonary resuscitation. The process of giving artificial breaths and manually pumping the heart muscle when a patient stops breathing and the heart stops beating.

**CVA**—Cerebrovascular accident. Also called a stroke, this is a blockage in the arteries in the brain or a hemorrhage into the brain that results in paralysis and, at times, difficulty speaking and changes in behavior.

**D&C**—Dilatation and curettage. A surgical procedure whereby the cervix is opened and suction is applied to the inner lining of the uterus.

**DDD**—Degenerative disk disease. A progressive disease whereby the disks (padding between the bones in the back) deteriorate.

**Decub**—Decubitus. A wound caused by pressure or poor circulation. Also referred to as an ulcer.

**DJD**—Degenerative joint disease. A progressive disease in which the joints deteriorate due to repetitive motion or the aging process.

**DM**—Diabetes mellitus. The body cannot convert sugars into energy.

**DVT**—Deep vein thrombosis. A blood clot deep in one of the veins in the body (usually in the legs).

**Emb.**—Embolus. Usually this term for a blood clot is preceded by the location of the blood clot. For example, pulmonary embolus is a blood clot in the lung.

**ESRD**—End stage renal disease. The final stage of a progressive and terminal kidney disease.

**Fx.**—Fracture. A break.

**HCVD**—Hypertensive cardiovascular disease. Heart disease caused by high blood pressure.

**Hemi**—Hemiplegic. Paralysis of one half of the body, the right side or the left side.

**HIV**—Human immunodeficiency virus. The virus that eventually leads to acquired immune deficiency syndrome (AIDS).

**HTN**—Hypertension (high blood pressure). A person has high blood pressure when the systolic pressure is 150 mm or more or when the diastolic pressure is 90 mm or more.

**Hypercalcemia**—High blood calcium. Leads to muscle cramps and can lead to irregular heart rhythms.

**Hyperglycemia**—High blood sugar. May mean that the patient is diabetic.

**Hypoglycemia**—Low blood sugar. May mean that the patient had too much insulin, did not have enough food, or exercised too much.

**Hypopotassemia**—Low blood potassium. Leads to muscle cramps and severe weakness.

**Hyst.**—Hysterectomy. Surgical removal of the uterus.

**IDDM**—Insulin dependent diabetes mellitus. The person with diabetes must have insulin injections to metabolize sugars.

**Lap**—Laparotomy. Surgical incision into the abdomen.

**LBBB**—Left bundle branch block. An irregular heart beat resulting from the left ventricle not getting an electrical message sent by the atria.

**LBP**—Low back pain. Pain in the low back area.

**Leukemia**—A blood disease with increased numbers of immature white blood cells that collect in the lymph nodes. Classified as either acute or chronic. Usually acute leukemia comes on suddenly and the patient dies unless he or she has a remission (the disease corrects itself for a period of time).

**MR**—Mental retardation. Poorly developed brain, which leads to difficulty with or an inability to learn.

**MR**—Mitral regurgitation. A backflow of blood into the left side of the heart due to a poorly closing valve between the atrium and ventricle.

**MRSA**—Methicillin resistant staph aureus. A serious bacteria that does not respond to antibiotic treatment.

**MS**—Mitral stenosis. A narrowing of the valve in the left side of the heart between the atrium and ventricle.

**MS**—Multiple sclerosis. A disease with lesions on the spinal cord that prevent normal movement. This disease becomes worse over time.

**MVA**—Motor vehicle accident. An accident with a vehicle (car, bus, motorcycle).

**MVR**—Mitral valve replacement. Surgical placement of an artificial valve between the left atrium and left ventricle.

**NIDDM**—Non–insulin dependent diabetes mellitus. The person with diabetes who does not need insulin to metabolize sugars. This person may need pills that decrease the amount of sugar in the blood or may control diabetes by eating an ADA diet.

**OBS**—Organic brain syndrome. A deterioration of brain tissue. Also called senility.

**OHS**—Open heart surgery. Heart surgery performed after opening the chest cavity.

**OM**—Otitis media. A middle ear infection. Symptoms might include severe pain, fever, and crying.

**Para.**—Paraplegic. Paralysis of the lower half of the body, usually as a result of a thoracic or lumbar spinal cord injury.

**PP**—Postpartum. After pregnancy.

**Quad.**—Quadraplegic. Paralysis of the four extremities (arms and legs), usually as a result of a cervical spinal cord injury.

**RBBB**—Right bundle branch block. An irregular heart beat resulting from the right ventricle not getting an electrical message sent by the atria.

**RSV**—Respiratory syncytial virus. An upper respiratory virus often seen in immunosuppressed and premature infants and children during the winter months. This can lead to lung complications such as pneumonia.

**SBE**—Subacute bacterial endocarditis. A bacterial infection of the lining of the heart.

**SBO**—Small bowel obstruction. A blockage in the small intestine. The patient develops irregular bowel movements, severe abdominal pain, and eventually vomiting.

**STD**—Sexually transmitted disease. Any disease transmitted through sexual relations. The virus or bacteria lives in the seminal and vaginal fluids that are transferred from one to another.

**T&A**—Tonsillectomy and adenoidectomy. Removal of the tonsils and adenoids (glandular tissue).

**Tachy**—Tachycardia. Rapid heart rate (100 beats per minute or more).

**TAH**—Total abdominal hysterectomy. The surgical removal of the uterus, ovaries, and cervix.

**TEF**—Tracheal esophageal fistula. An opening (which should not be present) leading from the esophagus (tube going into the stomach) to the trachea (windpipe leading to the lungs).

**TENS**—Transcutaneous electrical nerve stimulation. A battery-powered device that sends very fine electrical currents into the muscle to tire the muscle. Once the muscle becomes tired, it relaxes and pain is lessened.

**TF**—Tube feeding. Delivery method for liquid nutrition. Tube feedings are given through a tube passed through the nose and into the stomach or surgically implanted through the abdominal wall and into the stomach.

**THR**—Total hip replacement. A surgical placement of an artificial hip joint.

**TURB**—Transurethral resection of bladder. The surgical removal of bladder tissue done with instruments inserted into the urethra.

**TURP**—Transurethral resection of prostate. The surgical removal of some of the enlarged prostate gland tissue done with instruments inserted into the penis.

**UC**—Ulcerative colitis. An inflammatory disease of the large intestine. Symptoms include abdominal pain, severe diarrhea with mucus and blood at times, and loss of weight.

**URI**—Upper respiratory infection. A bacteria or virus that invades the upper respiratory tract (nose and throat).

**UTI**—Urinary tract infection. A bacteria or virus that invades the urinary tract (urethra and bladder).

**VD**—Venereal disease. Any disease transmitted through sexual relations. The virus or bacteria lives in the seminal and vaginal fluids that are transferred from one to another (same as sexually transmitted disease).

**VT**—Ventricular tachycardia. A rapid heart rate caused by the fast contractions of the ventricles.

## SYMBOLS

↑ —up, upper, elevate
↓ —down, lower
→ —right
← —left
↔ —transfers to and from
™ —trademark
✓ —check, done

≥ —greater than or equal to
≤ —less than or equal to
φ —no, none
= —equal to
< —less than
> —greater than
~ —approximately
@ —at, about
# —pound
' —hour
" —minutes
% —percent
/ —per
1° —primary
2° —secondary

Other symbols from your organization:

_____

_____

_____

_____

_____

## ABBREVIATIONS

### A

$\overline{a}$—before
A—achieved
aa—of each
AAROM—active assist range of motion
abd.—abdomen, abduction
ABT—antibiotic therapy
ac—before meals
Add.—adduction
ADL—activities of daily living
ad lib—as much as needed
Adm.—Admit
ak—above knee
am—morning
AMA—against medical advice
Amb.—ambulate, ambulatory, ambulation, ambulating
amp.—ampoule, amputee
amt.—amount

ant.—anterior (front)
appt.—appointment
Apt—apartment
AROM—active range of motion
art.—artery
ASAP—as soon as possible
assist—assistance
ausc.—ausculate, auscultation
Ax.—axillary

_____
_____
_____

### B

B—both, bilateral
B&B—bowel and bladder
Bereav.—bereavement
BID/bid—twice a day
bilat./bil.—bilateral (both sides)
Bl/Blk—black

Bld—blood
BLE—bilateral lower
  extremities
BLL—bilateral lower lobe
BM—bowel movement
BP—blood pressure
BR—Bedrest
bro.—brother
BRP—bathroom
  privileges
BS—breath/bowel sounds
BSC—bedside commode
BUE—bilateral upper
  extremities

_____
_____
_____

## C

c̄—with
C—centigrade
cal.—calories
cap.—capsule
CAT scan—computerized
  axial tomography scan
cath—catheter

Cath.—Catholic
cc—cubic centimeters
CC—chief complaint
Cerv.—cervical
Cl.—clear
Cldy—cloudy
cm—centimeter
CM—case manager
CNA—certified nurses'
  aide
CNS—central nervous
  system
c/o—complained of,
  complaints of
comp.—compound
cond.—condition
cont.—continue,
  continued
cop.—copious
CP—chest pain, cerebral
  palsy, cardiopulmonary
cpd.—compound
CPR—cardiopulmonary
  resuscitation
ct.—count
CTA—clear to
  auscultation

_____
_____
_____

**D**

D—diarrhea
d/c—discharge
del.—deliver
dgt./dgtr.—daughter
dia.—diameter
dil.—dilute
Dir.—director
DME—durable medical
  equipment
DO—doctor of osteopathy
DOE—dyspnea on
  exertion
DOPS—director of
  professional services
Dr.—doctor
dsg.—dressing
d/t—due to
Dx.—diagnosis

_____
_____
_____

**E**

EDC—expected date of
  confinement
e.g.—for example
elev.—elevate, elevated
elix.—elixer
et—and
ET—enterostomal
  therapist
emot.—emotions,
  emotional
eval.—evaluate
exc.—exercise

_____
_____
_____

**F**

F—Fahrenheit
F—fair
fath.—father
Fem.—female
FF—force fluids
fld(s)—fluid(s)
flex—flexion

FMD—family medical doctor
f/t—follow through
ft.—foot
f/u—follow-up
FWB—full weight bearing
FYI—for your information

_____

_____

_____

**G**

_____

_____

_____

**H**

H/A—headache
hemi—half
hgt—height
HHA—home health agency
hkp—housekeeping

HME—home medical equipment
Hmk—homemaker
HMO—health maintenance organization
HNV—has not voided
HOH—hard of hearing
hr.—hour
HR—heart rate
ht.—height
$H_2O$—water
Hyper—high
Hypo—low

_____

_____

_____

**I**

I—independent, intake, intact, instruct
IC—infection control
i.e.—that is
IM—intramuscular
imp.—impaired, impaction

in.—inches
inapp.—inappropriate
Inc.—incontinent
indef.—indefinite
indep—independent
I&O—intake and output
irreg.—irregular
IU—International Unit
IV—Intravenous

_____
_____
_____

### J

jt.—joint

_____
_____
_____

### K

_____
_____
_____

### L

l—liter
L/ Lt.—left
lac.—laceration
lat.—lateral
lax.—laxative
lb.—pound
LE—lower extremity
lg., lge.—large
LLE—left lower
    extremity
LLL—left lower lobe
LLQ—left lower quadrant
LMP—last menstrual
    period
LOA—level of activity
LOB—loss of balance
LOC—loss of
    consciousness, laxative
    of choice
LPN—licensed practical
    nurse
LS—lumbo-sacryl
LS—lung sounds

LUE—left upper
   extremity
LUL—left upper lobe
LUQ—left upper quadrant
LVN—licensed vocational
   nurse

_____

_____

_____

## M

MA—maximum assist
MA—medical assistance
max.—maximum
MC—Medicare
MD—medical doctor
med.—medicine
Med.—Medicare
mg.—milligram
ml—milliliter
mm—millimeter
mod.—moderate
MOM—Milk of
   Magnesia

$MOSO_4$—morphine
   sulfate
MSS—medical social
   service
MSW—medical social
   worker
MVI—multivitamins
MWB—minimal weight
   bearing

_____

_____

_____

## N

N—nausea
N/A—not applicable
NAS—no added salt
NB—newborn
neg.—negative
neuro.—neurological
NF—not found
NKA—no known
   allergies
no.—number

noct.—nocturnal, night
norm.—normal
NPO—nothing by mouth
NSS—normal saline
   solution
NWB—non-weight
   bearing

_____
_____
_____

## O

o—oral
Occ.—occasional
OD—right eye
OOB—out of bed
Op.—operation
OS—left eye
os—by mouth
OT—occupational
   therapist, occupational
   therapy
$O_2$—oxygen
OU—both eyes
oz—ounce

_____
_____
_____

## P

p̄—after
P—pulse
para—children
pc—after meals
PCH—personal care home
PCN—penicillin
PE—physical examination
PEARL—pupils equal and
   reactive to light
PEARLA—pupils equal
   and react to light and
   accommodation
Ped(s).—pediatric(s)
PI—performance
   improvement
pm—after noon
PMH—past medical
   history
po—by mouth
POA—power of attorney
POC—plan of care
poss.—possible
post—posterior, after
post op.—postoperative
PP—private pay,
   postpartum

PR—per rectum
prn—if needed
prob.—problem
PROM—passive range of
    motion
Prot.—Protestant
psych—psychiatric,
    psychological
pt.—patient
PT—protime, physical
    therapist, physical
    therapy
Pulse Ox—pulse oximetry

_____

_____

_____

## Q

q—every
q ___ h—every ___ hours
qd—every day
qh—every hour
qid—four times a day
qns—quantity not
    sufficient
qod—every other day
qow—every other week

qs—quantity sufficient
qt.—quart
quant.—quantity, quantify
qw—every week

_____

_____

_____

## R

R—right
R—respirations
RD—registered dietitian
re:—regarding
rec.—received,
    recommend
recur.—recurrent
ref.—referring, referral
regurg.—regurgitation
Rehab—rehabilitation
req.—request
resp.—respiration
RLE—right lower
    extremity
RLL—right lower lobe
RLQ—right lower
    quadrant
RML—right middle lobe

RN—registered nurse
r/o—rule out
ROM—range of motion
rot—rotation
RP—Rehabilitation
  Potential
RUE—right upper
  extremity
RUL—right upper lobe
Rupt.—rupture
Rt.—right
Rx—treatment, prescription

_____

_____

_____

## S

$\overline{s}$—without
S—sacral
sang.—sanguineous
sat.—saturated
SE—side effects
Sig.—signature
sl.—sublingual
sm.—small

SNF—skilled nursing
  facility
SNV—skilled nursing
  visit
SOB—shortness of breath
sol.—solution
S/P—status post
spec.—specimen
ss—one half
SS—salt substitute
SQ—subcutaneous
supp.—suppository
SV—supervisory visit
SW—social worker, social
  work
sympt.—symptoms

_____

_____

_____

## T

t—teaspoon
T—temperature,
  tablespoon
tab.—tablet

tachy—tachycardia
tbsp.—tablespoon
Tech.—Technician
TENS—transcutaneous
   electrical nerve
   stimulation
TF—tube feeding
Tib.—Tibia
tsp.—teaspoon
Tx.—treatment

_____

_____

_____

**U**

u—unit
UE—upper extremity
umb.—umbilicus
ung.—ointment
Uro.—urology
US—ultrasound

_____

_____

_____

**V**

V—vomiting
vag.—vaginal
vc—verbal cues
vd.—void
vit(s)—vitamin(s)
vo—verbal order
Vol.—volunteer
vs.—versus
v/s—vital signs
vss—vital signs stable

_____

_____

_____

**W**

$\bar{w}$—with
w—week
WBAT—weight bearing
   as tolerated
W/C—wheelchair
WE—weekend
WFL—within functional
   limits

wgt.—weight
wk—week
WNL—within normal
   limits
w/o—without
wt.—weight

_____
_____
_____

**X**

x—times

_____
_____
_____

**Y**

yo—year old
yr(s)—year(s)

_____
_____
_____

**Z**

z—dram

_____
_____
_____

# CHAPTER 3

# The Qualified Home Care Aide

## PREPARATION

Preparation to be a qualified home care aide begins with interest in this type of work. As with any other job, interested individuals should learn as much as possible about the position before interviewing or accepting a job. To learn about the job of home care aide:

- Talk with someone who is a home care aide.
- Ask a current aide a lot of questions:
  1. What are the day-to-day duties?
  2. Is the job hard? enjoyable? Why or why not?
  3. Is it comfortable going into someone's home to work?
  4. What happens if your car breaks down?
  5. Are the bosses helpful? nice? Why or why not?
  6. Can you make friends on this job?

- Ask the person conducting the interview:
  1. What are the expectations of the aide?
  2. Can you tell me about the organization? For example, how long have they been in business? What is their mission (written reason for being in business)? Who would you report to?
  3. How will you be trained for this job?
  4. Will the work be full or part time?
  5. What are the benefits and salary for this job?
- Review the job description and ask questions about anything that you do not understand. See the sample job description in Exhibit 3–1.

Make a good impression by preparing for the interview using the following guidelines:

- Take your best image with you to the interview.
  1. Wear neat and clean clothing.
  2. Wear limited jewelry (e.g., a watch, one set of small earrings, a necklace).
  3. Use only a small amount of perfume.

4. Do not chew gum.
5. Walk and sit up straight.
6. Remain calm.
7. Speak clearly and loudly enough to be heard.
8. Listen to what is being said, and respond to questions.

- Be ready to talk about
    1. any experience you have had to prepare you for a job as a home care aide
    2. why you want this job
    3. why they should hire you (talk about your good qualities, such as honesty, caring, compassion, ability to follow directions, etc.)
- Review and follow the information in the interview guide in Exhibit 3–2.

---

**Exhibit 3–1** Sample Job Description—Home Care Aide

| | |
|---|---|
| **Position Title**: <u>Home Care Aide</u><br>**Program Area**: <u>Clinical</u><br>**Date Approved**: _____<br>**Review Date/Initials**: _____<br><br>**Supervision:**<br>**Responsibilities** <u>X</u> No ___ Yes<br>**Nature of Supervision:** None<br>**Reports to:** Aide Supervisor | **Safety Equipment:**<br>Flexible goggles with side shields, antireflux respirator, and protective gowns, aprons, and gloves |

*continues*

**Exhibit 3–1**  continued

### Position Summary

Provides personal care to patients as delegated by a professional member of the patient care team. Responsible for paraprofessional aspects of care and patient safety. Functions under the overall supervision of the aide supervisor.

### Experience and Qualifications

High school graduate or GED preferred. Experience in caring for the geriatric population in a health care–related setting preferred. Must be able to communicate orally and in writing.

### Competency/Skill Requirements

CPR certified. Certified as a home health aide either through completion of an approved home health aide training course or through competency testing. Demonstrates good interpersonal relationship skills.

### Working Environment

Potentially unsafe and unsanitary home environments. Potential travel in inclement weather. Office environment.

### Position Physical Demands

Driving or riding in a motor vehicle, standing, sitting, walking, bending, reaching, and stretching. Lifting up to 50 pounds unassisted and up to 325 pounds using an assistive device.

### Key Responsibilities and Duties

1. Provides for the personal care needs of the patient as designated on the home health aide plan of care.
2. Reports changes in the patient's condition and needs in a timely fashion.
3. Documents care on the appropriate forms.

*continues*

**Exhibit 3–1**  continued

4. Submits to the organization completed documentation within established time parameters.
5. Performs all duties within the boundaries of the personal care policies and procedures.
6. Provides care to the patient with attention to the safety needs of the patient.
7. Performs household duties as designated by the care plan.
8. Uses equipment and supplies appropriately.
9. Revises workload and patient care assignments as requested by the aide supervisor.
10. Takes initiative in performance of assigned work, requiring minimal supervision.
11. Demonstrates a high degree of commitment to customer service and the provision of quality care.
12. Exhibits positive interpersonal oral and written skills.
13. Attends a minimum of 12 hours of continuing education/inservice each year.
14. Completes an annual skills assessment.
15. Participates in quality improvement activities and staff meetings.
16. Performs all other duties as requested or assigned.

I acknowledge receipt and understanding of this job description. I realize that this reflects a general list of responsibilities of the position, as well as a general description of the working environment and physical demands.

_____     _____

Signature                                              Date

*Source:* Reprinted with permission from ADVANTAGE Health Care Management Resources.

**Exhibit 3–2**  Interview Guide

---

**Before the Interview**

- Think about your past experience, your values, and your personality. Identify key points that are important to discuss during your interview, for example:
  - Do you have past experience as an aide?
  - Have you taken care of elderly grandparents or neighbors?
  - Have you done any volunteer work?
  - Would people who know you recommend you for this type of work? Why?
- Identify three individuals who will provide the agency with a reference about you and your work. If this is your first job, you can use the names of former teachers, clergy, or business-people. Take their addresses and phone numbers with you when you complete the application.
- Ask the identified individuals if they will offer a reference to the agency on your behalf.
- Complete the application neatly. Use a pen, not a pencil.
- If the agency asked you to complete an application without scheduling an appointment, obtain the name of the person responsible for hiring. Write and mail a short note identifying yourself and the fact that you completed an application and stating that you look forward to meeting with him or her.

**During the Interview**

- Dress in good clothes that are clean and in good repair. Do not wear jeans, sandals, or excessive jewelry or makeup.
- Do not chew gum, eat candy, or smoke during the interview.

---

*continues*

**Exhibit 3–2** continued

- Greet the interviewer with a smile and handshake. Your handshake should not feel like a raw fish nor should it be so forceful that it causes pain. Practice with a friend.
- Wait to be directed to a chair, and remember to use good posture.
- Refer to the interviewer as Mrs., Mr., or Ms. _____ unless asked to do otherwise.
- Be enthusiastic but not phony.
- Think about the question and plan your response before you talk. Try not to babble.
- After the interviewer has asked you about yourself and past experiences, ask any unanswered questions you may have.
- Thank the interviewer for his or her time, and find out when you can plan on hearing from the agency.

**After the Interview**

- Write a brief note thanking the interviewer for his or her time. Indicate in the note your interest in the position.

*Source:* Reprinted with permission from ADVANTAGE Health Care Management Resources.

# PROS AND CONS OF WORK AS A HOME CARE AIDE

It is wise to think about the good and not-so-good aspects of being a home care aide. However, what might be a good reason to become a home care aide for one person may be a not-so-good reason for another. The job has to be right for the individual. Working in home care means:

- You work as a guest in the patient's home.
- You have a chance to help those who cannot help themselves.
- You need to have special training and to be able to show that you know how to do the skills you will need.
- You need to travel from one house to another, seeing six or more patients a day.
- You work alone most of the time but can call the office for help if needed.
- You may not have close work friends, because you and the other aides work away from the office.
- You need to travel in all types of weather and road conditions.

To help you decide if the job is right for you, use Table 3–1. Read each item and check whether it is a "pro" (reason to take the job) or a "con" (reason not to take the job). More pro results indicate that the job may be right for you.

Thinking about these issues before accepting a job as a home care aide is smart. If you take a job and find that you do not like it, you waste your time and the agency's time. Some questions you may want to ask yourself are the following:

- How much do I depend on work for socializing? If you are a social person and have always had work

**Table 3–1** Job Analysis

| Category | Reason | Pro | Con |
| --- | --- | --- | --- |
| Home Care Aide as an Occupation | I (think I would) like the day-to-day duties of a home care aide. | | |
| | This type of work is (sounds) enjoyable. | | |
| | I like the idea of traveling from home to home. | | |
| | Reliable transportation from home to home is not a problem for me. | | |
| | Traveling in bad weather is not a problem. | | |
| Organization | This agency has a good reputation. | | |
| | I like this agency's mission (purpose) and values (how it does business). | | |
| | I felt comfortable with the people who interviewed me from this agency. | | |
| | This agency will train me for my job. | | |
| | The pay is good at this agency. | | |
| | The benefits are good at this agency. | | |
| | The hours are just what I want to work. | | |
| | There are opportunities for a job promotion or better benefits in this agency within a year. | | |

*Source:* Reprinted with permission from ADVANTAGE Health Care Management Resources.

friends that became your home friends, home care may seem very lonely to you. On the other hand, if you enjoy meeting and working with new people who are agency customers, you will probably like home care.

- If my car breaks down, how will I get to work? The patient needs care and so it is important to have a plan before you have a car problem. Some aides ask to borrow family members' cars if they have car problems.
- Do I like to drive or travel when there is snow on the road or I need to take a different road because of construction? Some aides find that they love to drive in the spring. There is nothing better than the fresh, spring air blowing in the car and the radio playing in the background. How will you feel when the day is cold and the roads are slippery from a winter storm?

Knowing what you are saying "yes" to is the first part of preparing to be a home care aide. The next part has to do with education.

## EDUCATION

To become a home care aide, you must be educated. The rules vary from state to state and agency to agency. Some require that you have a high school education, while others require a certain number of years of schooling. It is important that you be able to:

- Read English.
- Write short sentences in English.
- Report to and take direction from someone else.
- Follow directions.
- Use common sense.

In addition to formal education, you have to be trained to do the skills that you will need to do with the patients. Before being allowed to work as a home care aide, you will need to pass a test showing that you understand and are able to perform the skills.

## SKILL ASSESSMENT

You will need to be able to do the following skills:

- Talk with patients and their family members and caregivers (helpers).
- Introduce yourself to patients in their home.
- Respect the rights of patients while caring for them in their homes.
- Assist or completely bathe a patient who is in bed, at the sink, in the tub, or in the shower.
- Shave the male patient's face and female's patient's legs and underarms.

- Shampoo the patient's hair in bed, at the sink, in the tub, or in the shower.
- Clean and file nails.
- Provide skin care and massages.
- Assist the patient with undressing and dressing.
- Assist the patient with changing positions (e.g., from lying to sitting, sitting to standing).
- Assist the patient with walking using a cane, walker, crutch, or you for support.
- Assist the patient with going to the bathroom or using a bedpan or urinal.
- Move the patient with a lift device or wheelchair.
- Take the patient's blood pressure, temperature, and pulse.
- Assist with range of motion and other exercises.
- Prepare meals.
- Provide simple house cleaning (e.g., dishes, dusting, vacuuming).
- Follow guidelines for personal and patient safety, such as infection control and good body mechanics.

These skills are part of the training that you need to become a home care aide. Some agencies and states want you to attend and pass a 75-hour training course, while others will accept past work training or life experience as long as you can pass a written test and demonstrate the skills. The skills course will be discussed in detail later.

## ATTITUDE ASSESSMENT

People have different attitudes about life and work. Attitudes are sometimes called "good" or "bad." There are reasons for attitudes that people have. Home care agencies find that hiring aides with certain attitudes seems to work best for the agency, aide, and patients and their families. Attitudes that agencies look for include the following:

- sympathetic and caring about the sick
- willingness to help others
- mature thought process
- able to deal effectively with the demands of the job (HCFA, 1995)
- self-confidence
- positive outlook with a cheery nature
- able to make decisions

Additionally, the following values are important to the agency and patients:

- *Dependability.* You work when you are scheduled.
- *Reliability.* You do what you say you will do.
- *Dedication.* You give a full hour of work for an hour of pay.
- *Patience.* You do not rush the patient through the care.

- *Gentleness.* You are not abrupt in the care you provide.
- *Good listening skills.* You not only hear the words, you connect with the patient and respond in a meaningful way.
- *Honesty.* You provide the ordered care and report events as they actually happened.
- *Caring.* You pay attention to the patient and treat him or her as a special person.

If given a choice between someone with a good attitude and values and someone with good skills, employers often hire the person with the good attitude and values. Skills can be taught, but attitudes are more difficult to change.

## TRAINING COURSE

Formal home care aide training programs must meet the requirements of the federal government's (Health Care Financing Administration) regulation listed in the HIM 11 (HCFA, 1995), including the following:

- The training must take place over 75 hours.
- The 75-hour course must include 16 hours of practice in a laboratory setting.
- A registered nurse, or other professional under the direction of a registered nurse, must teach the course.

- The registered nurse must have two years of experience as a registered nurse, one year of experience in a home care setting, and six months of experience supervising 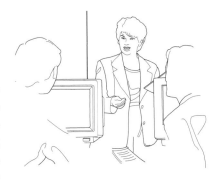 home care aides. (At the time of writing, some changes regarding the requirements for the person teaching the course are pending.)

The regulations were a little confusing when they were first written. The federal government wanted people to take the course and pass a test to become a home care aide, but the regulations, as written, require taking the course and/or passing a test. This means that agencies can make choices about the training they want their home care aides to have, if any. If the state has requirements, the agency must follow the state law if state requirements are more strict than the federal law.

Information that must be covered in a training course includes

- communication
- observation, reporting, and documentation of patient status

- taking, reading, and recording temperature, pulse, and respiration
- basic infection control procedures
- clean, safe environment maintenance
- recognizing emergencies and knowing what to do in an emergency
- physical, emotional, and developmental needs of the populations served and ways to work with them, including the need to respect the patient and his or her property and privacy
- respect of privacy and property
- safe and appropriate patient hygiene and grooming, including
  1. bed bath
  2. sponge, tub, or shower bath
  3. shampoo in sink, tub, or bed
  4. nail and skin care
  5. oral hygiene
  6. toileting and elimination
- safe transfer techniques and ambulation
- normal range of motion and positioning
- adequate nutrition and fluid intake
- any other task that the agency may choose to have the aide perform

## Competencies

To become a home care aide, the aide must pass a competency evaluation of all of the skills listed above. If the aide does not pass one of the skills, the aide cannot provide that type of care unsupervised. Aides are permitted to test again on the skills that they have not passed.

## Clinical Practicum

A clinical practicum allows aides to practice their skills in a clinical setting. For Medicare certification, the skills must be observed on a live person and not a mannequin. Most of the clinical practicum is done with classmates, but some skills, such as urinal use, bedpan use, and bathing private areas, are done in the patient's home under the supervision of the trainer.

## LEARNING NEW SKILLS AND COMPETENCIES

Taking tests and being observed by someone else can be unnerving. Many people being trained as home care aides have not been in a formal class setting for some time. They are adults. If you are an adult, you should be aware of the following characteristics of adult learners:

- They have a brief attention span (about 15–18 minutes). This means that they need frequent changes of subject matter and breaks.
- They learn by doing. This means that rather than just listening to the training, you need to be able to practice.
- They may have lost their confidence in learning and testing. This means that the trainer should offer a lot of compliments. Learners should work at recognizing what has been learned rather than focusing on what they have failed to learn.
- They have more lifetime experiences from which they can draw comparisons. This means that the learner should have more to discuss and share while learning.
- They are afraid to talk in class because they may be wrong. Try it! Your trainer will be very supportive and appreciative of what you have to share. The rest of the class may learn something from you!

The following suggestions can help you when taking tests or being observed by your supervisor:

- Prepare by reading and practicing.
- Relax.
- Ignore the fact that you are being observed (without appearing rude).

- If you cannot remember, put your pen down, close your eyes, and focus on relaxing. As you relax, the information will come back.
- Talk with the patient if you are being observed.

## ONGOING EDUCATION

Medicare requires that you have at least 12 hours of ongoing education every year to keep your certification as a home care aide. This education is often called inservice education, presentations, seminars, or lectures. The education does not have to be a formal presentation. It can be a self-study guide or prepared education information that you can read, such as *The Home Health Aide Educator,* published by ADVANTAGE Health Care Management Resources Press. Whether you attend a lecture, read a prepared inservice, or go to a seminar, it is very important that you write down the topic and number of hours spent in ongoing education to prove that you did in fact have 12 hours of inservice. Failure to attend 12 hours of inservice during any one year means that you must take the certification test and clinical practicum over again.

Medicare-approved agencies have to show their surveyor written proof that aides attended 12 hours of inservice during any one year. In some states the aide is required to mail a list of all education attended. In any case, you should be very aware of your total inservice hours and help track the inservice education so that you are able to maintain your certification.

Agencies have different processes to give inservice education and to document it (write it down) in preparation for their surveyor's visit. Educational methods include

- requiring that each home care aide attend one hour per month or three hours per quarter
- using videotaped inservices for those who missed the inservice or about unusual topics or topics required annually by law (e.g., worker safety, universal precautions)
- providing written self-learning educational materials
- offering 15 minutes of education prior to weekly aide meetings
- offering one full-day and then one half-day seminar annually

Education documentation methods include the following:

- A secretary documents the inservice for each person in attendance.
- The aide documents each inservice on a card in the office.
- A paper is passed around at each inservice and home care aides sign in.

## HOME CARE AIDE DOs AND DON'Ts

### Do

- Follow the rules of the agency (e.g., dress code, absentee reporting).
- Ask for help if you do not know something or do not understand a procedure.
- Seek clarification of information about the patient that you do not know.
- Call your supervisor if in doubt.
- Report to work on time.
- Document accurate and honest information in the patient's clinical record and on your time cards.
- Attend ongoing education.
- Follow through with requests for administrative needs, such as copies of certifications, health care exams, and so forth.
- Practice universal precautions to control infections. (These are discussed in detail in Chapter 7.)
- Think about your surroundings in the car, on the street, and in the patient's home, and practice personal safety measures. (These are discussed in detail in Chapter 7.)
- Listen to the patients with interest.
- Consider both the patient and the caregiver (e.g., husband, wife, friend) as your customers.

- Call your supervisor or the patient's nurse with information about changes in the patient and new problems.
- Document and turn in your paperwork on time.
- Offer some possible solutions whenever you have a complaint or concern to share with your supervisor.
- Recognize that you are not the boss and the agency does not owe you a living.

## Do Not

- Do not treat patients roughly.
- Do not yell at patients or coworkers.
- Do not use profanity.
- Do not wear excessive or dangling jewelry such as necklaces or earrings. Confused patients can grab onto these items and tear your earlobes or choke you.
- Do not call in sick unless you are sick.
- Do not rush through your patient care.
- Do not smoke in the patient's home.
- Do not borrow or take anything that does not belong to you.
- Do not talk about the patient or the patient's condition with anyone but your supervisor and others at work who have a need to know.

# CHAPTER 4

# People Skills

## INTRODUCTION

Mahatma Gandhi is quoted as saying "You must not lose faith in humanity. Humanity is an ocean; if a few drops of the ocean are dirty, the ocean does not become dirty" (*Reader's Digest Great Encyclopedic Dictionary,* 1975, p. 2037). People's relationships and interactions with others are not always perfect, but in the whole sea of people, there really are very few who "dirty the waters."

As a home care aide, the skill of getting along with people is very important. Coworkers, supervisors, patients, and families are a few of the people with whom you will interact every day you are on the job. Each person has a different background and different life experiences that make up who he or she is. Every person sees the world of today through eyes of yesterday. You do not have to become psychic to read people's minds; you just need to be open to the possibilities that exist—in personalities, in cultures, in backgrounds, and in your day-to-day activities as you work and play.

## UNDERSTANDING PEOPLE'S COMMUNICATION STYLES AND BEHAVIORS

According to the president of the American Listening Association, there are four levels of communication:

1. Small talk is that which is done when people first meet or greet each other, for example:
   - Great weather, isn't it?
   - Have you watched the Olympics this week?
   - Isn't the sky a deep blue today?

   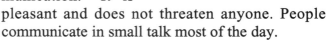

   This type of communication is considered "surface communication." It is pleasant and does not threaten anyone. People communicate in small talk most of the day.
2. Cathartic communication occurs when the speaker is emotional about something. The emotions could

be anger or happiness. Cathartic communication means that the person who is talking tells everything to the listener and "gets it all out." If you have ever had a bad day and spent your entire dinner talking about it, you engaged in cathartic communication.

3. Information exchange is another type of communication. Facts and steps in a process or procedure are the subject matter of information exchange. A newlywed calling home to Mom to find out how long the chicken needs to be in the oven takes part in information exchange. A home care aide being oriented to a new patient is exchanging information with the nurse.

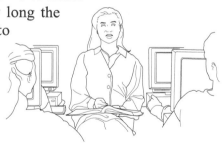

4. Finally, persuasive communication is the fourth level of communicating. The purpose of this style

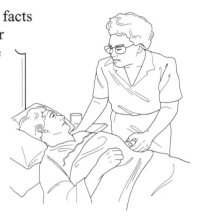

is to provide enough facts so that the listener forms the same opinion as the message sender. A patient may want to use persuasive communication to achieve his or her request for a tub bath today even though the aide care plan specifies that a bed bath be given.

## COMMUNICATION GUIDELINES

Communication requires at least two people: someone who sends a message and someone who receives the message. Figure 4–1 diagrams the communication loop. The sender forms the words that are sent based on personal past experience and education. This is during the formulation period of the message indicated by the X on the left side of the figure. If the sender is a home care aide who tried to make a suggestion and was criticized, he or she may choose a different style or method to communicate the suggestion. Once the sender gives the message, the receiver interprets it. The receiver thinks about the message and translates the words and the manner in which the message was sent based

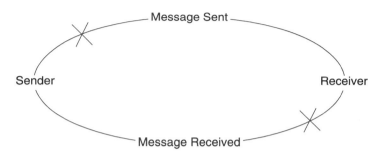

**Figure 4–1**  The Communication Loop

---

on his or her own past experiences. This interpretation occurs at the point of time noted by the X on the right side of the figure.

Given the fact that every person is different and has experienced different situations in life, it is not hard to understand why people fail in their communications 85 percent of the time. It isn't that we don't try—we just receive the message differently than the sender intended. Some guidelines for the sender and receiver follow.

### Sender

- Be at ease when you communicate to:
  1. Put the receiver at ease.
  2. Encourage two-way communication.
  3. Help identify individual concerns and pressures.

- Allow the listener time to speak freely and without interruption. In the long run this saves time that would be wasted in repeat communications. It also provides you with an additional perspective of the issue.

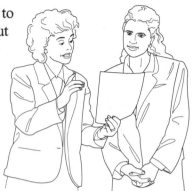

- Clarify any miscommunications that have occurred.
- Seek input from the listener if not offered.
- Avoid jargon, and recognize the variations in the meanings of words from generation to generation (e.g., "rocks," "partner," "gay").
- Present the most important points early in the encounter—don't save the best for last.
- Clearly state what is expected or needed.
  1. Summarize key points, deadlines, and any confusing aspects.
  2. Plan for a follow-up if needed.
  3. Describe what you mean.
  4. Make a statement instead of asking a question.
- Consider your timing and your approach.
  1. What just happened in your day?
  2. What just happened in your receiver's day?

    3. What aspects of the receiver's world need to be considered?

    4. What happened to the receiver in the past that formed the receiver's personality and how he or she will interpret your message?

- Do not be judgmental.
- Do not embellish the message.
- Recognize that as the sender you have the responsibility to be clear and concise and to elicit feedback that clarifies that what you wanted the listener to receive is what the listener received.

## Receiver

- Breathe. In addition to being a vital function to sustain life, breathing helps you to relax and look interested instead of upset.
- Listen intently.

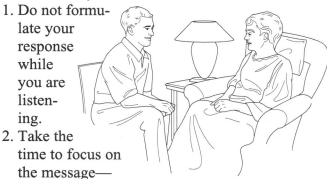

    1. Do not formulate your response while you are listening.

    2. Take the time to focus on the message—

both what is being said and the meaning behind what is being said.
- Clarify what you do not understand.
- Acknowledge what you have heard, including the valid points.
- Take time to contemplate what you have heard before responding.
- Consider your style of communication and the self-corrective actions you might want to make before responding.

## MODES OF COMMUNICATION

Communication can be oral, nonverbal, or written. Nonverbal messages that people send, often without realizing it, are the most difficult mode of communication. Think about a teacher you had in school who had "that look." As a child, your mother or father may have had "that look" also. It may have been a stare, a tightened jaw, or a slight twist of the neck. The person did not have to say a word, but you received a strong message that what you did was not acceptable. Nonverbals are fun to watch. The next time there is a serious issue to be discussed at home or at work, be aware of what people are doing. Folded arms and frowns communicate anger or disagreement. Sitting and leaning slightly toward the group shows interest in what is being said.

## PERSONALITY TRAITS

Psychiatrists have studied personalities and identified similar traits. There are tests available (e.g., Myers-Briggs and Kiersey-Bates) to identify the traits in individuals' personalities. The results are always interesting and usually give individuals some insight into differences between themselves and their coworkers and families. If anything, it helps to explain that there is no right or wrong personality, just different personalities. Learning about the people you live or work with helps to explain why some people "drive you crazy" and others are "just great." Some personality traits are described below.

### Extroversion versus Introversion

Most of the population is extroverted. These individuals are sociable and enjoy parties and taking part in outside activities. Extroverts process information quickly. Sometimes they are inaccurate but confident in their position. Once the information is processed, extroverts verbalize much of what they are thinking. A smaller portion of the population is introverted. These individuals tire easily in social settings. They prefer quiet events with a few people rather than a party with a lot of people. They are private in their thoughts and prefer a few, close friends. Introverts process information more slowly. They think about the situation or issue for hours or days and then develop their plan of action. To extroverts, the introvert may appear indecisive and slow at problem solving. They are neither—just different.

### Sensing versus Intuition

Most people fall into the sensing category. These individuals work hard to get a job done. They are considered the sensible ones in the crowd, using past experiences to solve today's problems. On the other end of the spectrum are the intuitive thinkers. When faced with a decision, these people get a strong hunch. They are sometimes considered to be airy because they are very imaginative and think of possibilities that the sensors just would not consider. These are the people who join "think tanks." They are imaginative and futuristic.

### Thinking versus Feeling

The population is split 50/50 with this trait. Thinkers feel more comfortable with a policy or law to guide them. They are more prone to think in opposites: right versus wrong, black versus white. Others note that thinkers are interested in what they are doing, not in who they are doing it with. Feelers are people persons. They connect with others and are very personable. Feelers justify why the policy or law was not appropriate due to the special circumstances surrounding the situation.

## Judging versus Perceiving

Again, the population is split with this trait. Judging people do just that—they judge the situation or person and make a decision. They have opinions and do not like to waste time deciding what they already know. Perceivers are open to alternatives. They believe that if they wait, the information and answer will come to them. They would prefer to postpone a decision until the answer is more clear. Unlike the judges, the perceivers do not pay attention to deadlines (Myers and Briggs, 1991; Keirsey and Bates, 1984).

If this topic is of interest to you and you want to read more about personalities and take a test to learn about your personality, the book *Please Understand Me Character & Temperament Types* by Keirsey and Bates (1984) is recommended.

## BEHAVIORS

In addition to personalities, people differ in behaviors. Behaviors, unlike traits, are not always good. For example, sometimes people may be aggressive, assertive, or passive. Home care aides need to recognize these behaviors and learn how to work with (or around) them.

### Aggressive Behavior

#### *Types*

- Wanting control of everything
- Not liking to delegate
- Putting people down in private or in public
- Calling people names that are not polite
- Acting superior to others
- Strongly pushing others to have the same beliefs
- Being confrontational or direct in approach
- Placing blame on others
- Being manipulative at times
- Thinking that they are okay but others have problems
- Working all the time because they think no one else can do it as well
- Making demeaning comments, sch as "Look at what you did again"

### *Dealing with Aggressive Behavior*

If individuals are angry:

- Give them time to talk and calm down.
- Listen to their point of view. State that you understand what they are saying without agreeing with their view.
- Ask questions to get the facts.
- Do not counterattack.
- Stay calm. Be friendly.
- Say the person's name frequently.
- Give facts to support your position.
- Use a firm tone of voice.
- Interrupt if necessary.

If the behavior is out of control:

- Firmly tell them to stop or sit down.
- Stand up to gain control.
- Indicate that you want to discuss the situation when they are in control.
- Postpone the discussion, if necessary.

If they are being sarcastic:

- Ask them to explain what they mean by the remark.
- Let them know that you do not appreciate their sarcasm.
- Use a calm and controlled voice.

## Passive Behavior

### *Types*

- Keeping thoughts, opinions, and feelings inside
- Preferring to wait for someone else to take the lead
- Losing sight of who they are
- Trying to make others happy and having no time left for themselves
- Being easy prey for those with aggressive behavior
- Being prone to depression, even suicide
- Believing that they are not okay and that, in fact, nothing is really okay nor will it be

### *Dealing with Passive Behavior*

- Listen attentively when these people start to talk.
- Let them know that they are appreciated.
- Ask questions to get the facts.
- Ask open-ended questions, such as "what do you think about it?"
- Offer your opinion after they have had a chance to tell you their thoughts.
- Do not agree with ongoing whining and complaining. State your experiences if they differ from theirs.

**Passive Aggressive Behavior**

*Types*

- Enjoying gossip
- Preferring to get even rather than get mad
- Using guilt to control
- Making "poor me" statements
- Blaming others

*Dealing with Passive Aggressive Behavior*

- Banter with them using a playful tone of voice.
- Ask questions in an unemotional tone of voice.
- Problem solve, if indicated.

**Assertive Behavior**

The behaviors described above are not good behaviors. Assertive behavior is preferred. Assertive behavior leads to healthy self-esteem and problem solving to develop a win-win situation. Characteristics of assertive behavior are as follows (Shaffer, 1994; Scholtes, P., et al., 1991; Development Dimensions International, 1987):

- Using communication that is honest and direct
- Showing respect for others and being sensitive not only to the needs of others but to one's own needs
- Believing that everyone is okay

## LEARNING TO LIKE YOURSELF

It is rather common to have behaviors or traits that you do not like in yourself. Identifying those issues and trying to make personal changes are signs of maturity. Some steps you can take to lead to self-acceptance include the following:

- Take time for yourself.
- Ask someone close to you to describe your good qualities.
- Look at yourself through the eyes of a friend.
- Talk with a professional.
- Describe yourself, using every letter of the alphabet to start a word.
- Commit to be kind to yourself.

## LEARNING TO ACCEPT OTHERS

Hopefully through learning and understanding personality traits and behaviors you can begin to look at your world differently. Just because other people have traits that are different does not mean that they are bad or wrong. They are just different. In their book *Please Understand Me Character & Temperament Types*, Keirsey and Bates begin with the following insightful excerpt:*

> *If I do not want what you want, please try not to tell me that my want is wrong.*
>
> *Or if I believe other than you, at least pause before you correct my view.*
>
> *Or if my emotion is less than yours, or more, given the same circumstances, try not to ask me to feel more strongly or weakly.*
>
> *Or yet if I act, or fail to act, in the manner of your design for action, let me be.*
>
> *I do not, for the moment at least, ask you to understand me. That will come only when you are willing to give up changing me into a copy of you.*
>
> *I may be your spouse, your parent, your off-spring, your friend, or your colleague. If you will allow me any of my own wants, or emotions, or beliefs, or actions, then you open yourself, so that*

---

*Source:* Reprinted with permission from D. Keirsey and M. Bates, *Please Understand Me Character & Temperament Types,* © 1984, Prometheus Nemesis Book Company.

*some day these ways of mine might not seem so
wrong and might finally appear to you as right—
for me. To put up with me is the first step to understanding me. Not that you embrace my ways
as right for you, but that you are no longer irri-
tated or disappointed with me for my seeming
waywardness. And in understanding me you
might come to prize my differences from you,
and, far from seeking to change me, preserve and
even nurture those differences.*

## HAVING PROBLEMS GETTING ALONG WITH YOUR SUPERVISOR?*

Supervisors do not always say and do things the way
that staff think they should. Sometimes a supervisor asks
staff to do things differently than they want to do them.
Sometimes staff might think that the supervisor is just
being mean or trying to cause trouble for them. This does
not *feel* good. In fact, it makes them feel like they do not
want to listen or cooperate with the supervisor. You
might not always agree with your supervisor, but it is
important to understand why.

---

*Source:* Reprinted with permission from *The Home Health
Aide Educator,* Vol. 1, No. 3, ADVANTAGE Health Care
Management Resources Press.

Remember that if you think about your life—the fun times, sad times, and events that happened to you (and are happening right now)—you understand how

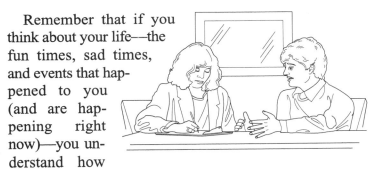

those things have made you who you are today. Most of what you think and do makes sense to you. It is "normal." You are behaving the way "everybody" else does.

As it turns out, what is okay for you may be not okay for other people, including your supervisor. In fact, other people may say things or do things that seem odd or "wrong." In reality, no one is always right or always wrong. There are just differences between people. By trying to "walk a mile in your supervisor's shoes" (or the shoes of your coworker, friend, or relative), you should think about the following:

- What kind of experiences did that person have in life?
- What kind of stress is the person under at work? (For example, what are your supervisor's responsibilities? What does his or her supervisor demand?)
- Does your supervisor act differently because of his or her culture or position at work?

- If you met your supervisor on the street, would you like him or her?
- Do you really think your supervisor does not want to get along with people?

Full-time workers spend one third of their day at work. People would rather get along than have problems, and your supervisor probably agrees with this statement. Here are 11 steps you can take to help make the situation better*:

1. Ask to meet with your supervisor, in private, when he or she has time.
2. Be kind. Act the way you want your supervisor to act with you.
3. Begin by saying something kind to your supervisor. For example, thank him or her for doing something nice or just for taking the time to meet with you.
4. Describe the work relationship you want with your supervisor.
5. Tell your supervisor about the problems you are having. Give examples.
6. Describe how you feel when this happens.
7. Ask your supervisor to help you with the problem.
8. Be prepared to discuss some solutions with your supervisor.

---

*Source:* Reprinted with permission from *The Home Health Aide Educator,* 1998, ADVANTAGE Health Care Management Resources Press.

9. Listen to what your supervisor has to say.
10. If there is something that you can do to change the situation, work on it.
11. Thank your supervisor for helping you with the problem.

Usually these steps lead to resolution. Many times, problems arise because people do not communicate well with each other. Communicating in home health care is difficult because aides are often out in the patient's home and supervisors are often back in the office. This makes understanding each other harder. The suggested straight-forward, 11-step approach should work and allow you to feel in control of your position.

## GAMES PEOPLE PLAY

Believe it or not, people are not always what they seem to be. Dr. Eric Berne, a noted psychiatrist and originator of transactional analysis, outlined several games that people play in their relationships with others in his book *Games People Play*. Transactional analysis is the study of commu-nications: what message was sent, how it was received, and the response to the message. Berne explains that games are a way of life. They are played in life, in marriages, in the boardroom, at parties, and at work. Sometimes the outcome of the game is good, but other times the outcome is hurtful to someone involved. It is therefore helpful to recognize games and their purposes in order to avoid using games when the expected outcome is harmful. You might recognize some of the games that Berne identified and find that you play one of the roles.

**Game 1—The Alcoholic** (Berne, 1964)

This is a game that may be playing in your personal life or the lives of some of the patients under your care. It is important to understand that patients (and even co-workers) might be in one of these roles.

Roles: "It," "Persecuter," "Rescuer," "Patsy"

Casting:

| Role | Part | Behavior/Comments |
|------|------|-------------------|
| "It" | The alcoholic | Full circle: drinks and is ostracized, doesn't drink and is complemented, goes back to drinking |
| "Persecuter" | The spouse of the alcoholic | "Poor me" attitude<br>Somewhat of a martyr |
| "Rescuer" | A child, friend, or spouse | Intervenes to "make everything right" |
| "Patsy" | A spouse, child, or friend | Acts as the parent by helping the alcoholic to undress or keep appointments ("the helper") |

Plays: Can you identify the role being played?

- The alcoholic is quick to offer a friend a drink. Once the friend accepts, the alcoholic has to drink with the friend because "it's only right."

- The alcoholic father drank too much and the son hides the fact from Mom to keep peace in the family.
- The local bartender allows the alcoholic to run up a tab. He is such a nice guy.
- The husband helps his alcoholic wife up the stairs and into bed after a party.

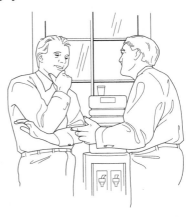

## Game 2—Ain't It Awful
(Berne, 1964)

This game is common to the workplace.
Roles: "Us–Them" or "Me–You"
Casting:

| Role | Part | Behavior/Comments |
|------|------|-------------------|
| "Us" | One part of the whole: staff/ management/ aides, etc. | Meet somewhere (lunch, in the hall, at the patient's home) and complain and relay stories leading to the conclusion that "they" are really being awful to "us" |
| "Them" | The other side or another part of the whole | "They" may just be doing their job or perhaps they are playing games with "us" |

Plays: Can you identify the role being played?

- You overhear two nurses talking at a desk in the office. They are whispering about the new policies just handed down from their supervisor. One starts to complain about how unrealistic the expectations are just as another nurse enters and relates a story about the supervisor's nasty comment about the new policy.
- The aide is on time and committed to doing a good job with her patients. She attends a staff meeting and hears that the professional staff think the aides should be more productive.

**Game 3—Now I Got You, You Son of a Gun**
(Berne, 1964)

Roles: "Me," "You"
Casting:

| Role | Part | Behavior/Comments |
|------|------|-------------------|
| "Me" | Someone who perceives that he or she has been wronged | Does not address the situation with "you." Instead, waits until a good opportunity to pay back "you." The goal is to hurt "you." |
| "You" | The other person | Knowingly or unknowingly has hurt "me." May apologize appropriately or not recognize the hurt he or she has inflicted on "me," thus there may be no change in behavior. |

Plays: Can you identify the role being played?

- The supervisor evaluates the aide as (only) meeting the standards in the job description.
- Three months later the aide is asked to give input about her supervisor's performance for her evaluation. The aide makes negative comments that are untrue. The supervisor receives a poor evaluation.

## Game 4—Stupid (Berne, 1964)

This is another game played in the workplace.
Roles: "Stupid," "Other"
Casting:

| Role | Part | Behavior/Comments |
|------|------|-------------------|
| "Stupid" | Anyone desiring less work | This person just cannot learn what he or she is supposed to do and jokes about being stupid and incapable. |
| "Other" | A boss or coworker | Laughs with "stupid" and then lets "stupid" get by without learning what is expected ("After all, the poor person is too stupid to learn!") |

Plays: Can you identify the role being played?

- The new secretary disconnects callers whenever she is asked to transfer a call. This becomes the office joke.

- The secretary's boss changes her job description. She no longer needs to answer the phone and transfer calls.

### Game 5—Let's You and Him Fight (Berne, 1964)

This is another game played in the workplace.
Roles: "Perpetrator," "You," "Him/Her"
Casting:

| Role | Part | Behavior/Comments |
|------|------|-------------------|
| "Perpetrator" | Any worker | This individual figures out the angles, identifies something that he or she doesn't like and leads you to believe that "him/her" doesn't like it so that you and "him/her" battle out the problem. |
| "You" | You | You believe "perpetrator" and address the issue with "him/her" only to discover that you have been duped. |
| "Him/Her" | A third person (possibly the victim in *Now I Got You, You Son of a Gun!*) | Pulled into a situation, this person knows that he or she is out on a limb but may be unsure as to who is responsible or why it happened. |

Plays: Can you identify the role being played?

- Jane, the aide, is called in to talk to her boss. When she meets with her boss, she finds out that her friend, Susie, told her boss that Jane was not pleased with the scheduler's attitude. Her boss is upset because she thought that Jane felt comfortable coming directly to her with problems. In reality, Susie met with Jane just yesterday to complain about the scheduler and Jane made one comment about one small problem she had. Jane did not think this was a major problem until now.
- Susie was really upset with Nancy, the scheduler. She talked with all of the aides and the only aide who had anything negative to say was Jane. When Susie saw her boss, she told her that Jane was really upset with Nancy and might quit.
- The aide supervisor always cared about the happiness of the aides. She heard that Jane, one of her best aides, was upset.

## DEALING WITH IMPROVEMENT

No one is perfect. With age come maturity and wisdom. As wisdom is gained, people may identify changes that could lead to personal improvements. Sometimes supervisors guide and help staff to understand the improvements that are needed, and other times staff guide themselves. In some agencies, yearly goals for improvement are a routine part of the evaluation process. Some guidelines for improvement plans are as follows:

- Improvement plans should be developed at routine intervals. If they are not done as part of your evaluation you might want to personally evaluate yourself for opportunities for improvement every year around your birthday.
- They can include both personal and work-related goals.
- They should be developed with your supervisor's input.
- Goals should be specific and measurable, for example:
  1. to take 15 minutes out of the day for myself beginning tomorrow
  2. to arrive at work on time 100 percent of the time over the next three months
- Improvement should be maintained by
  1. tracking performance
  2. attending ongoing employee developmental sessions as planned

## Formal Call for Action from Supervisor

Work-related issues can lead to a formal counseling session with your supervisor. Generally, these fall into three categories of concerns:

1. Quantity of work:
   - Employee does not complete work as assigned.
   - Employee is unable to make as many visits as needed to meet the budget.
   - Documentation is turned in late.
2. Quality of work:
   - Employee visits too many patients in one day in order to take the next day off.
   - Patients complain that the employee provided rushed and incomplete care.
   - Payroll reporting is falsified.
   - Clinical record audits reflect poor documentation or the lack of coordinated care planning.
3. Poor work habits (Developmental Dimensions, International, 1987):
   - The employee frequently arrives to work 10–15 minutes late.
   - The aide takes more than a half hour for lunch.
   - The employee takes too many breaks.
   - The employee interrupts others trying to work.

When supervisors identify a concern, they should follow a process to make certain that they have all the facts. Exhibit 4–1 identifies the process steps that a supervisor follows before taking action. Most organizations have a formal process regarding how to proceed. For example, the organization may begin with a verbal warning and then use a written warning, suspension, and finally termination. Agencies can skip any of these steps, depending on the severity of the problem.

## SELF ASSESSMENT APPLICATIONS

Use the assessment in Exhibits 4–2 and 4–3 to assist you with self-understanding.

---

**Exhibit 4–1** Fact-Finding Process for Formal Employee Counseling

1. Incident
2. Previous Infractions
3. Degree of Infraction—Establish Penalty
4. Due Process
5. Disciplinary Action
6. Meeting Preparation
7. Summary Documentation
8. Outline of Situation
9. Potential Actions
10. Behavioral Response

*Source:* Reprinted from B. Gingerich and D. Ondeck, *Human Resource Manual for Home Health Care,* © 1997, Aspen Publishers, Inc.

**Exhibit 4–2** Communication Inhibitors

| SELF-ANALYSIS COMMUNICATION TOOL | | | | |
|---|---|---|---|---|
| Do you . . . (check the appropriate boxes and add up the numbers) | | | | |
| *Rarely* | | | | *Frequently* |
| Not listen | 1 | 2 | 3 | 4 | 5 |
| Talk too much | 1 | 2 | 3 | 4 | 5 |
| Talk too little | 1 | 2 | 3 | 4 | 5 |
| Give mixed messages | 1 | 2 | 3 | 4 | 5 |
| Misinterpret | 1 | 2 | 3 | 4 | 5 |
| Use poor timing | 1 | 2 | 3 | 4 | 5 |
| Avoid eye contact | 1 | 2 | 3 | 4 | 5 |
| Interrupt | 1 | 2 | 3 | 4 | 5 |
| Lecture | 1 | 2 | 3 | 4 | 5 |
| Praise falsely | 1 | 2 | 3 | 4 | 5 |
| Subtotal | | | | | |
| TOTAL | | | | | |

*Scoring Interpretation*
Under 11—Great Communicator
11–20—Good Informer
21–30—Borderline Talker
31–40—Mixed Messages
Over 40—Bad News

*Source:* Reprinted with permission from ADVANTAGE Health Care Management Resources.

**Exhibit 4–3** Communication Enhancers

| SELF-ANALYSIS COMMUNICATION TOOL | | | | | |
|---|---|---|---|---|---|
| Do you . . . (check the appropriate boxes and add up the numbers) | | | | | |
| | *Rarely* | | | | *Frequently* |
| Clarify | 1 | 2 | 3 | 4 | 5 |
| Use simple directions | 1 | 2 | 3 | 4 | 5 |
| Make eye contact | 1 | 2 | 3 | 4 | 5 |
| Give feedback | 1 | 2 | 3 | 4 | 5 |
| Stay open-minded | 1 | 2 | 3 | 4 | 5 |
| Listen attentively | 1 | 2 | 3 | 4 | 5 |
| Use pauses/silence | 1 | 2 | 3 | 4 | 5 |
| Choose the setting | 1 | 2 | 3 | 4 | 5 |
| Use new ideas | 1 | 2 | 3 | 4 | 5 |
| Use open-ended questions | 1 | 2 | 3 | 4 | 5 |
| Subtotal | | | | | |
| TOTAL | | | | | |

*Scoring Interpretation*
Over 40—Great Communicator
30–39—Good Informer
20–29—Borderline Talker
11–19—Mixed Messages
Under 11—Bad News

*Source:* Reprinted with permission from ADVANTAGE Health Care Management Resources.

# CHAPTER 5

# The Patient/Family Care Unit

## INTRODUCTION

Caring for patients, especially in their own homes, involves not only the patient but also the patient's family and informal caregivers. By the time patients seek help from an outside agency, they usually have had some needs met by friends and family members. When agency workers, including the home care aide, first enter the patient's home, they enter as a guest. If you are that home care aide, you must understand that a strong bond often exists between the patient and the family/caregivers. You are the outsider and need to adjust. (This is much different than caring for a patient in the hospital or nursing home. In these facilities, there is a structure with procedures and processes. The patient needs to fit into those procedures and processes.) This chapter provides information that will help you to understand the patient and tips for becoming a part of the patient/family bond that exists. There are some actions that you can take that will make you very valuable in the eyes of these customers (patients and family/caregivers).

## PATIENT RIGHTS

Beginning in 1973 and continuing over the years, the federal government, accrediting bodies, and health care associations identified the rights of patients and adopted these rights as standards. Health care workers are responsible for knowing, understanding, and respecting these rights, which include the following:

1. *The patient has the right to receive care in a considerate and respectful manner.* This basic patient right means that the home care aide must be considerate (thoughtful and kind to others) and respectful (work without taking over or intruding) of the patient.

2. *The patient has the right to receive information from health care workers in an understandable, relevant, and current manner.* Health care workers are physicians, nurses, therapists, dietitians, and aides. This right means that all of these workers must give patients the most up-to-date (current) information about their care and their condition (relevant because it is about them) in words that they can understand (understandable). It does *not* mean that the home care aide can educate patients about their diagnosis. It does not mean that the nurse can educate patients about the best exercise program. It does

mean that each worker should educate the patient about the activities that that worker performs. As a home care aide, you can educate the patient and family/caregiver about bathing or skin care or turning. Each worker must be careful to give only the information that he or she is educated to give.

3. *The patient has the right to be given the opportunity to discuss and request information related to the specific procedures and treatments, the risks involved, the possible length of recuperation, and the medically reasonable alternatives to care, including risks and benefits of each.* As a home care aide, you can comply with this right by explaining to the patient what you are about to do, such as turning, shampooing in bed, or any other task. If the patient asks, you must discuss other ways of performing the care. For example, patients with severe pain may want to move themselves to their side rather than have you and their spouse turn them. This should be permitted as long as it is safe and possible.

4. *The patient has the right to know the identity of all caregivers as well as the experience level of each.* You need to introduce yourself to your patients. If they want additional information about your experience, you must tell them. Remember, even if this is your first patient, you should tell them that you are certified to work as a home care aide. Explain what that means (e.g., you took a test, attended classes).

5. *The patient has the right to contribute to decisions related to his or her plan of care prior to and concurrent with the course of treatment.* As a home care aide, you need to allow the patient to make some decisions about his or her care. For instance, if a patient does not want you to shave him, you must follow his wishes. If a patient does not want to have visiting nurses or therapists coming to his home, his wishes must be honored.

6. *The patient has the right to refuse a recommended treatment or plan of care to the extent permitted by law and to be informed of the medical consequences of such action. In the case of refusal, the patient is entitled to other appropriate care and services that the organization provides or assistance with transfer of service to another organization.* The patient can refuse any portion of the care or all of the care, and you must follow his or her wishes. Patients can refuse to take medicine, refuse to go to the hospital, or refuse your entrance into their home. Remember to follow patient rights numbers two and three listed above. If the patient refuses care, you must give him or her information about the risks of that refusal. If a Medicare patient is refusing to have a bath but wants you to empty the trash and dust the living room, Medicare will not pay for that care. The patient has a right to be told that he or she runs the risk of having the aide care discontinued.

7. *The patient has the right to receive information about and to formulate advance directives.* All adult patients entering home health care must be informed about advance directives. Advance directives include living wills and selecting someone as a medical power of attorney. Living wills are written and signed guidelines to help the physician make medical decisions if the patient is unable to make those decisions because of a physical or mental condition. They are signed by the person while in good health or in advance of the need for decision making. In another kind of advance directive, the patient chooses someone who will make medical decisions when he or she is unable to do so because of a physical or mental condition. The chosen person becomes the patient's medical power of attorney. This is not the same as a legal power of attorney. The person with medical power of attorney cannot make legal decisions for the patient (e.g., sign checks, give permission for purchases).

8. *The patient has a right to expect that advance directives will be followed.* Once the patient has signed an advance directive, health care workers must follow the instructions. This means that if the patient does not want to be put on a ventilator if there is no chance of living a quality life, the physician cannot put the patient on a ventilator if he or she believes that there is no chance of the patient living a quality life. Some confusion exists about

advance directives from a legal view. In the above example, how does the physician really know that the patient has no chance of living a quality life? As a result, some states have declared advance directives to be guidelines and given physicians legal permission to use them as guidelines and not a legal statement that must be followed.

Check with your agency to find out what your role is with advance directives and add it here.

My role is _____

_____

_____

_____

9. *The patient has the right to every consideration of privacy.* For example, when bathing patients, you must keep as much of their body covered as possible. Other actions you can take to ensure privacy are to keep the door closed and to ask them if they want you to leave the room (if it is safe) while they use the toilet, bedpan, or urinal.

10. *The patient has the right to expect that all communications and records pertaining to care will be treated in confidence.* This right means that you are not allowed to share information about any patient. Sometimes people might ask you for information because they are

friends and are concerned. You are not allowed to say anything about the patient. If faced with this situation, you can say, "I'm sorry. I am not permitted to discuss anything about other people." You can also acknowledge that you understand their concern and suggest that they call the person.

Be aware that you could share information without meaning to by

- leaving your paperwork unprotected, thereby allowing interested people to read about the patient
- posting the aide care plan on the refrigerator where any visitor in the home can read the care being provided
- having the patient sign a timesheet that has other patient names on it

11. *The patient has the right to review his or her records and to have the information explained or interpreted as necessary, except when restricted by law.* If a patient asks to look at his or her record, you should call your supervisor to find out what process the patient is to follow. If there are no laws in the state, the agency may still have procedures to follow.

12. *The patient has the right to be informed about expected outcomes to treatment.* Patients should be told that as a result of the home care aide service they will be clean and their sheets will be changed. This is usually

done by the person admitting the patient to the agency. You can also explain the purpose of your visit to follow this regulation.

13. *The patient has the right to be informed about barriers to care.* Barriers to care are found on occasion. They may be financial, environmental, physical, or care related. For example, the agency may have only one occupational therapist, who is on a two-week vacation. If the physician wants the patient to have occupational therapy, the patient (and physician) must be informed that the therapy will not be available for two weeks. If the patient lives in an unsafe environment and the agency will not send anyone there after dark, the patient needs to be told that in-home care is not available after dark.

## PATIENT RESPONSIBILITIES

The Joint Commission on Accreditation of Healthcare Organizations (Joint Commission) is an organization that sets rules for quality in health care. Agencies ask the Joint Commission to visit and evaluate how well they work in relation to these rules. One of these rules is explaining patient responsibilities to them when they receive health care. The reason for patient responsibilities is to make sure that the agency has the most current information about the patient and has a good chance of meeting the needs and expectations of the patient. These are not a law, but many agencies list patient responsibilities. You may want to check with your supervisor about your organization's patient responsibilities.

In my agency, patients

- ❏ are given information about their responsibilities
- ❏ are not given information about their responsibilities

If they are given responsibilities, they may include the following:

1. *The patient is responsible for giving complete and accurate health information to the organization. Should condition changes occur, it is the patient's responsibility to provide the information as soon as possible.* This responsibility protects the health care workers and the patient. If the patient has (or gets) an infectious disease, the patient must notify the agency. Should this happen, the health care workers can take extra precautions or go to their physician for treatment, if needed. The agency will make changes in the plan for caring for the patient that will give the patient the best care available.

2. *The patient is responsible for providing accurate financial information to the organization.* The patient must tell the organization when his or her insurance changes or runs out. This allows the patient and agency time to find another payment source or make new plans for care.

3. *The patient is responsible for assisting in the revision of the plan for care.* Patients must give the agency staff information about their condition and any changes in medicine, physician appointments, and care. This means that patients are an important part of their health care team and have both input and a responsibility to the team for their care.

4. *The patient is responsible for notifying the organization's staff when he or she is unable to understand instructions or treatment directions.* Patients must tell the agency when they are confused or do not understand what they have been told. This relates to the discussion about communications in Chapter 4. As a home care aide, you may think that you are speaking very clearly, but if the patient does not understand, it is his or her responsibility to tell you so that you can reword it.

5. *The patient is responsible for notifying the organization of any changes in telephone numbers or residence.* It only takes one time of not being able to contact or find a patient to understand this responsibility. If patients do not notify the agency when they move, then the agency cannot give them the care that they need. Most agencies have a process to follow if they cannot find a patient. Some suggestions are provided in the next section of this chapter.

6. *The patient is responsible for notifying the organization of any concerns or problems related to care received.*

## WHAT TO DO IF . . .

### There Is No Answer to Your Knock at the Patient's Door

1. Try another door or a window in the room where the patient often stays.
2. Telephone the patient.
3. Call your supervisor for direction.
4. Call the patient's emergency contact if directed to do so by your supervisor.

### The Patient Has No Respiration or Heart Beat

1. Assess for the signs of death:
   - no response to vigorous shaking and loud shouting
   - no breathing
   - no pulse
   - eyelids slightly or fully open (possible sign)
   - mouth slightly open (possible sign)
   - loss of control of urine and/or feces (Do not take time to check for this.)
2. If the patient is to be resuscitated and you are trained to perform CPR:
   - Begin CPR.
   - Yell for help.

- Ask someone to call an ambulance (911).
- In the absence of help, call an ambulance but do so quickly so you can resume CPR.
- Continue CPR until help arrives, a physician tells you to stop, or you can no longer continue.
- Call your supervisor.
3. If the patient is *not* to be resuscitated:
    - Check the patient for a pulse and respirations.
    - Provide support to the family/caregivers.
    - Notify your supervisor for direction.

## The Patient Refuses Care

1. Ask the patient why.
2. Explain the risks of refusing care, if any.
3. Call your supervisor.

## The Patient and/or Family/Caregiver Is Upset about the Care

1. Remain calm.
2. Ask them to explain their concerns.
3. If you think they have a valid point, offer an apology, and tell them that you appreciate their honesty and that you will not repeat the behavior.
4. Ask them if they want you to contact your supervisor for a replacement.
5. Inform your supervisor of the situation.

## GROWTH AND DEVELOPMENT

Life is one stage after another. It is rather interesting to watch people grow from infancy through old adulthood. Although each person is an individual, some common age-related characteristics exist. Working with patients in all age groups makes a home care aide's day interesting. To better understand what patients of all ages are experiencing, home care aides should know some of the more common characteristics.

### The Infant

Table 5–1 contains a developmental guide that details the milestones in the development process for infants from newborn through the age of one year. Remember, each infant is different, but development generally falls within the time frame given. Premature infants will be behind by the number of months of prematurity but usually will "catch up" by age 3. For example Jill was born 4 months premature, she is now 10 months old. To obtain Jill's "adjusted developmental age," subtract 4 from 10 and you obtain 6. Jill should have the abilities of a six-month-old.

### The Child and Adolescent

Children are very interesting people. They are full of energy and curiosity about everything. Children have a

**Table 5–1** Infant Developmental Milestones

| Age | Ability |
| --- | --- |
| One month | Lifts head occasionally, but unsteady in ability to maintain control |
| | Able to turn head side to side when lying on belly |
| | Stares at surroundings |
| | Able to identify bright objects and facial presence if directly in front |
| | Smiles |
| | Cries when uncomfortable |
| | Makes small throaty sounds |
| Two months | Able to hold head up |
| | Able to lift head and part of chest when lying on belly |
| | Follows moving light |
| | Smiles socially |
| | Listens to voices |
| | Develops different cries for different needs |
| Three months | Holds head up and steady |
| | Able to hold head and chest up through arm support when lying on belly |
| | Plays with hands and objects |
| | Looks toward objects within a limited range of vision |
| | Blinks when object threatens eyes |

*continues*

**Table 5–1** continued

| Age | Ability |
|---|---|
| | Laughs |
| | Makes more vocal sounds |
| | Cries less |
| | Recognizes people seen frequently |
| Four months | Able to hold head and chest at a 90° angle when on belly |
| | Able to turn from back to side |
| | Likes to be propped up and attempts to support self |
| | Recognizes objects |
| | Plays with and tastes objects |
| | Laughs and smiles in response to others |
| | Coos and gurgles socially |
| | Loves attention |
| Five months | Sits with little support |
| | Reaches for objects in an extended field of vision |
| | Demonstrates increased "talking" when happy or sad |
| Six months | Sits briefly without support |
| | Able to pull self up into a sitting position |
| | Jumps up and down in one place with feet fixed on the floor |

*continues*

**Table 5–1** continued

| Age | Ability |
| --- | --- |
| | Turns from front to back to front |
| | Bangs objects |
| | Moves backward when in a sitting position |
| | Uses more syllables with babbling |
| | Recognizes people who are not seen daily |
| Seven months | Attempts to sit up when lying down, but only able to lift head |
| | Moves toys between hands |
| | Rolls easily |
| | Changes emotional moods quickly from laughing to crying |
| | Cries and makes "mmm" sound |
| Eight months | Able to sit alone steadily |
| | Demonstrates coordination between hands and eyes |
| | Greets strangers with bashfulness or crying |
| | Appears apprehensive around strangers |
| | Reaches out for hugs and cuddles |
| | Shows continued speech development |
| Nine months | Able to put nipple in and out of mouth |
| | Uses one hand more than the other |
| | Crawls |

*continues*

**Table 5–1** continued

| Age | Ability |
| --- | --- |
| | Begins to imitate sounds |
| | Cries when scolded |
| 10 months | Makes stepping movements when held upright |
| | Walks sideways with furniture support |
| | Feeds self "finger foods" |
| | Able to say a word or two |
| | Enjoys playing pat-a-cake and peek-a-boo |
| 11 months | Stands erect with adult support |
| | Evidences increased ability to control eye-hand coordination |
| | Shows increased verbalization |
| 12 months | Stands alone |
| | Walks with help |
| | Able to drink from a cup |
| | Helps while being dressed |
| | Demonstrates increased vocabulary |
| | Shows more emotions, such as jealousy, anger, affection, frustration |
| | Sees the world only from a self-centered perspective. |

*Source:* Reprinted from B. Gingerich and D. Ondeck, *Clinical Pathways for the Multidisciplinary Home Care Team, 1995–1998,* © Aspen Publishers, Inc.

very short attention span (less than one minute), and therefore getting a message across is best done with humor and brevity. Adolescents are very different from children. Their needs and emotions often change. It is very important to provide care for the adolescent that acknowledges that the adolescent is approaching adulthood. Table 5–2 provides information about growth and development from toddler through adolescent years.

**Table 5–2** Childhood and Adolescence

| Stage | Activities |
|---|---|
| Toddler (age 1–3) | Prefers to do things for self |
| | Self-centered |
| | In early stage, may be afraid of strangers and become anxious when familiar people (Mommy, Daddy) leave |
| | Speech development |
| | Negative (e.g., favorite word is "no") |
| | Knows a few body parts |
| | Uses "mine" to describe toys and objects |
| | Refers to self by name |
| | Curious about surroundings |
| | Explores cupboards and drawers |

*continues*

**Table 5–2** continued

| Stage | Activities |
| --- | --- |
| Preschool (age 3–5) | Helpful<br>Able to follow simple instructions<br>Knows most body parts<br>Is afraid of physical injury or hurt (Ahmann, 1996, p. 62)<br>Can stand on one foot (3 years) and progresses to skipping (5 years)<br>Fine motor skills beginning to develop<br>Identifies with adult of the same sex |
| School age (age 6–12)<br>  Early (6–9) | Increasing interests outside the home<br>Strong food preferences; gobbles meals<br>Extremely active; hard to sit still<br>Learns skills such as swimming and riding a bicycle<br>Susceptible to illnesses<br>Selects own clothes<br>Is messy<br>Needs to be reminded to pick up room |

*continues*

**Table 5–2** continued

| Stage | Activities |
| --- | --- |
| Middle (9–12) | Allergies may become apparent |
| | Prone to minor accidents |
| | Girls have a growth spurt |
| | Needs increased amounts of rest |
| | Poor posture |
| | Loves conversations |
| | Can become rebellious with family standards |
| | Strong influence of a best friend |
| Adolescent (age 13–19) Early (13–14) | Rapid physical growth |
| | Crushes on teachers or famous people |
| | Time of group identity formation |
| | Dresses, speaks, and acts like peers |
| | Close friendships with same sex |
| | Talking to friends a popular activity |
| | Wide mood swings |
| | Sports-centered interests—boys |
| | Clothes and makeup interests—girls |
| Middle (13–17) | Attains physical maturity |
| | Beginning of abstract thinking |

continues

**Table 5–2** continued

| Stage | Activities |
|-------|------------|
| | Idealism |
| | Self-centered |
| | Conflicts with parents over independence |
| | Acceptance by peers of great importance |
| | Fears rejection |
| | Creative period |
| | Withdraws when upset or feelings are hurt |
| | Outside jobs for spending money begin |
| Late (17–19) | Adult physical features finalized |
| | Views problems comprehensively |
| | Begins shaping life goals and tasks |
| | Self-esteem stabilized |
| | Forms attachments and stable relationships |
| | Decreasing importance of peer groups |
| | Dating partner and male-female relationships emerge |
| | Decrease of creative imagination |
| | Stabilization of mood swings and emotions |

*Source:* Reprinted with permission from ADVANTAGE Health Care Management Resources.

## The Aging Process

As people age, natural changes occur from a social, spiritual, physical, and psychological perspective. Adulthood is divided into many stages. These stages also contain certain tasks and activities that are common to most individuals within the stage.

The elderly patient has special physical and psychosocial needs. This patient has entered the last stage of life. The elderly have increasing physical health problems, and as they grow older, their friends and family die, leaving them isolated and lonely. As a result, many elderly can be easily deceived by people with bad intentions.

Table 5–3 describes the expected changes, tasks, and activities of adulthood. As a home care aide, you can help the elderly by doing the little things that count.

**Table 5–3** Adulthood

| Stage | Activities |
| --- | --- |
| Early adult years (approximately ages 17–22) | Leaves behind the adolescent world<br>Identifies one's position in an adult world<br>Becomes more self-sufficient<br>Separation from family<br>May make life-long commitment through marriage |

*continues*

**Table 5–3** continued

| Stage | Activities |
|---|---|
| Adult entry/ Young adult (approximately ages 23–29) | Autonomy from parents established<br>Chooses and prepares for a career/ occupation<br>Develops marital or other form of relationship<br>Personal lifestyle and philosophy developed<br>Participates in citizen behaviors<br>Transitions fully into the adult role<br>Settles into an occupation<br>Marriage and children<br>Commitments made but are change-able during this phase<br>Becomes responsible |
| Settling down period (ages 30–39) | Life takes on more of a serious tone<br>Settles into a structured routine<br>Begins to show signs of gray hair |
| Middlescence I (30–50—spans settling down and middle adulthood) | Evaluates career with personal value system<br>Helps younger persons to become integrated to job<br>Enhances intimacy with spouse/ significant other<br>A few deep friendships |

*continues*

**Table 5–3** continued

| Stage | Activities |
|---|---|
| | Assists elders through later years of life |
| | Responsible: social, civic, organization, community |
| | Maintains and improves home |
| | Secures other types of property |
| | Leisure time: more creative and satisfying activities |
| Middle adulthood (ages 40–59) | Pursues mentoring and parental relationships |
| | May realize career goals and dreams |
| | Continued graying of hair |
| | Some wrinkling of facial skin (e.g., forehead, crows feet) |
| Middlescence II (51–65 spans middle adulthood and older adult) | Flexible views maintained |
| | Current on science, news, politics and culture |
| | Mutually supportive relationships with children or other members of the next generation |
| | Adapting to signs and symptoms of aging |
| | Adjusting to loss of relationships |

*continues*

**Table 5–3** continued

| Stage | Activities |
|-------|-----------|
| | Assisting aging parents through last stages of life |
| | Planning for retirement and perhaps another career |
| Older adult (approximately ages 60–69) | Trunk becomes shorter |
| | Transition to retirement |
| | Continued signs of aging (graying, wrinkles) |
| | Sensory loss begins (hearing, vision) |
| Elderly (approximately 70–84) | Loss of muscle mass |
| | Continued sensory loss |
| | Skin becomes thin and frail |
| | More prone to infections |
| | Begins review of life experiences |
| | May have system deterioration |
| | Prone to forgetfulness |
| Aging changes | Delayed gastric emptying |
| | Impaired absorption |
| | Decreased appetite |
| | Incontinence |
| | Constipation |
| | Diminished emotions |
| | Less adaptability |

*continues*

**Table 5–3** continued

| Stage | Activities |
|-------|-----------|
| | Narrowing of interests |
| | Balding, "agespots" |
| | Blemishes more frequent |
| | Decreased ability to focus on new objects |
| | Increased difficulty with colors |
| Old-Old (85 and older) | Preparation for death |
| | Progressive decline with all systems |
| | Quiet, less active lifestyles |
| | Experiences sense of loss from death of friends and family |

*Source:* Reprinted with permission from ADVANTAGE Health Care Management Resources.

## THE PATIENT AND FAMILY/CAREGIVER UNIT

The family has changed over the past several decades. The family of yesterday had

- multiple children
- extended family members living together and helping others through illness
- mothers who stayed home to care for the children and home

- fathers who worked to support the family financially
- illness and diseases without cures, leading to more deaths and death at all ages

Today's family often has:

- one parent as the head of the household
- working parents
- no parental figure at home during work hours to care for others
- relatives living in different cities and states
- fewer children
- more choices of places to get help for sick relatives
- fewer ties to the family's cultural background

Various individuals can be the patient's family/caregiver unit. People who are included may be parents, spouse (husband or wife), children (daughters and sons), friends, neighbors, and even extended family members such as cousins, great aunts, and so on. Figures 5–1 through 5–3 show the concentric circles of support and closeness for three different patients.

In example one (Figure 5–1), Mr. and Mrs. Glass occupy the center circle. They have always been able to count on each other and rarely ask others for help. In fact, it is hard for them to ask for help. They want to be independent. In a pinch they can always call their son or daughter, who live close by, or their next door neighbor, Mr. Pope. If the problem is serious, they can call on their

**Mr. Glass**

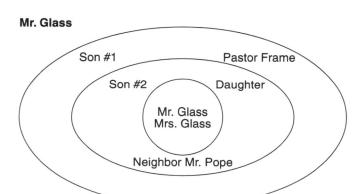

**Figure 5–1** Patient and Family/Caregiver Units—Example 1

oldest son who lives in a bordering city. He loves his parents but has personal problems with an ill child and failing marriage. Pastor Frame has always offered to help the Glasses, but they would hesitate to call on him unless there were a real need. The circles of support and closeness are set up over years of behaviors. Mr. and Mrs. Glass are very nice people, and most likely others would gladly help them out and occupy their center circle if they would only allow it to happen.

In example two (Figure 5–2), Miss Finch has several people in her inner circle. They include her sisters, who live with her. The sisters have numerous close cousins with children and grandchildren who always stop in to

**Miss Finch**

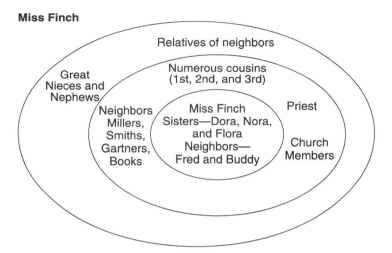

**Figure 5–2** Patient and Family/Caregiver Units—Example 2

bring vegetables from the garden or homemade soup. The local priest and several members of the church also stop by to help. Over the summer the church takes care of the sisters' lawn and gardening. Miss Finch and her sisters have a long history with the community, and offers of help come from relatives of neighbors and great nieces and nephews. Probably all of these people would help on a moment's notice, but Miss Finch has her priorities of who she feels the most comfortable calling for help.

In example three (Figure 5–3) Mrs. Martin lives alone. Her only contact with the outside world is a great nephew who lives on the opposite coast.

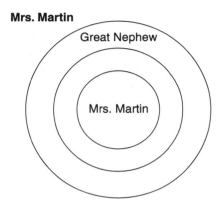

**Figure 5–3** Patient and Family/Caregiver Units—Example 3

These stories and examples show:

- Patients have different levels of comfort with asking for help.
- Patients sometimes have more help than they want to admit or use.
- Patients sometimes have no one to count on but outside help, such as the home care agency.

## SPECIAL PATIENT POPULATION NEEDS

### The Mentally Ill Population

Mental health is the ability to function in society. People with good mental health are able to cope with the stresses of day-to-day living. Patients diagnosed with mental illnesses lose their ability to cope with day-to-day situations. It is difficult for these patients to identify when they began to have coping problems but easy for them to identify the point when they could no longer cope.

As a home care aide you may identify some behaviors used to cope with day-to-day stress. Patients with poor mental health depend on various behaviors to get them through the day, including

- aggression—abusive and controlling behavior
- denial—refusing to accept reality
- depression—feeling saddened by reality
- projection—blaming others for problems
- rationalization—making excuses to make the behavior seem appropriate
- repression—putting stressful thoughts out of mind
- regression—returning to a less mature time in life

If you see any of these behaviors or other behavioral changes in your patients, be sure to report them to your supervisor.

**Prenatal Population**

These patients are expecting a baby. They may have acute or chronic health care problems or problem pregnancies. Home health care provided to this population is usually for:

- skilled care related to the acute/chronic condition
- nursing assessments of the pregnancy and the status of the unborn baby
- home care aide/homemaker care of the home while the patient is confined to bed
- child care aide services to care for children while the patient rests in bed

The prenatal home care patient should:

- eat a well-balanced diet
- avoid stress
- get out of bed only for the amount of time permitted by the physician
- get at least eight hours of sleep per day
- listen to what her body is telling her (e.g., if tired, sleep; if hungry, eat)

## The Postpartum Population

As with the prenatal population, postpartum home care visits are made for:

- skilled care related to the acute/chronic condition
- nursing assessments of the woman after delivery of a baby
- nursing assessments of the newborn
- education by the nurse regarding care of the mother and newborn

- home care aide/homemaker care of the home while the patient is recovering from a difficult pregnancy or birth
- child care aide services to care for the newborn and older children while the new mother rests in bed

The postpartum patient needs:

- adequate amounts of rest
- a well-balanced diet
- time for incision care (e.g., sitz bath)
- time for mild exercise (e.g., walking)

## WHAT ARE THE PATIENT'S NEEDS?

The lives and support available to Mr. Glass, Miss Finch, and Mrs. Martin (Figures 5–1 through 5–3) illustrate that different patients and family/caregiver units have very different needs of the home care agency. As a home care aide, you can help patients with individual needs that are marked with an asterisk (*) in the following list:

1. Social:
   - friendships
   - conversations with others*
   - getting out of the house
   - celebrating family occasions and holidays
2. Physical:
   - assistance with activities of daily living*

- elimination of the source of pain and suffering
- maintenance of personal hygiene*

3. Financial: The home care aide should not get involved with anything in the financial category. If the patient has financial needs, the aide should report this to his or her supervisor. Financial needs can include:
   - paying bills
   - banking
   - home maintenance (e.g., lawn care, roof replacements)
   - paying large bills (e.g., taxes, insurance)
   - high cost of health care (e.g., physicians, medications)

4. Emotional:
   - support for varied concerns*
   - talk therapy from a professional

## COMMON PATIENT EMOTIONS

Patients with long-term (chronic) or sudden (acute) illnesses often have the following concerns and emotions:

- fear of the unknown
- concern about who will care for them when they can no longer be independent
- ongoing pain and disability
- sense of loss

- depressed mood due to the loss of function
- guilt for depending on others
- anger at body for failing the patient
- financial concerns

As a home care aide, you can help by recognizing these concerns and emotions and talking with the patient. Once you have developed a good relationship with the patient, you can begin a conversation with "I sense that you are concerned about something. Can I help?" This opening lets patients know that if they want, they can talk with you. Sometimes patients need to talk but do not want to worry their family. Talking with their home care aide is better for them. Support the patient. If patients share any serious concerns (e.g., they are thinking of killing themselves), tell them that you are very concerned, and share this information with your supervisor as soon as possible.

## HOW DO I ANTICIPATE PATIENT NEEDS WITHOUT BEING TOLD?

Patients and families appreciate helpers who do not have to be told (or asked) to do each thing that needs to be done. Anticipating the patient's needs comes with time on the job. When you arrive at the patient's home for the first time:

- Review the care plan and discuss the care with the patient.
- Find out where the supplies are located (basins, soap, towels, lotion, etc.).
- Ask permission to get supplies out without help in upcoming visits.
- Ask the patient to tell you what he or she likes or wants. For example, does the patient use soap for face washing? Does he or she want lotion on the back?

By asking the patient on the first visit, you can get an idea of what the patient's needs will be in the future. You might want to make some notes for yourself to help you remember at the next visit. If you are going to be off, leave some notes for the next aide or call the aide to discuss the patient's desires. You may need to take a day off from time to time, but the patient should not suffer because you deserve some time away.

You will make your patients happy when you can look at them and know what they need. If they look uncomfortable, they probably are uncomfortable. Think about it—if you were in that position, what would you want? If that was your grandmother or grandfather, what would you want the home care aide to do to help him or her? If you had this disease, what would you be thinking? Try to put yourself in the place of the patient, and then you will be able to anticipate needs.

## WHAT INFORMATION NEEDS TO BE REPORTED TO THE SUPERVISOR?

As a home care aide, you act as a liaison (a go-between) between the agency and the patient and family/caregiver, the agency's customers. Report the following to your supervisor:

- any concerns the patient voices about the agency or agency staff
- any patient refusal of care
- any changes in the patient's condition
- anything that you do not understand
- any concerns you have about the patient
- any patient request for changes in the care plan
- any signs of abuse or neglect

## SIGNS OF ABUSE AND NEGLECT

Patient abuse and neglect happen every day somewhere, and for different reasons. Do not judge the abuser or neglectful person as a bad person. He or she may be very well intentioned but have difficulty coping with the situation. This may be a cry for more help. If you have any concerns that the patient may be abused or neglected, the best thing you can do to help is to contact your supervisor. Exhibit 5–1 lists some signs of abuse and neglect to help you to identify them with your patients.

**Exhibit 5–1**  Signs of Patient Abuse and Neglect

**PATIENT ABUSE**
**Physical**
- Bruises
- Scratches
- Burns
- Expressed fear of someone
- Suddenly becomes quiet when the abuser enters the room

**Emotional**
- Yelling and cursing
- Demeaning comments

**Financial**
- Stealing
- Keeping the patient in the home to cash and use his or her Social Security/pension checks for household bills

**All Types**
- Refusal to talk about the abusive person

**PATIENT NEGLECT**
- Patient has no food in the house.
- Patient is in same clothing as when the home care aide last visited (days ago).
- Patient is in same position as when home care worker last visited.
- Patient has no medications.
- Patient has signs of dehydration.
- Patient is lying in a soiled bed.

*continues*

**Exhibit 5–1** continued

> - Patient is left lying in bed without any stimulation from others (e.g., no one talks with the patient).
> - Patient has skin rashes
> - Patient has bedsores
>
> *Source:* Reprinted with permission from ADVANTAGE Health Care Management Resources.

## GETTING ALONG WITH THE PATIENT AND FAMILY/CAREGIVER UNIT

There is a common saying among lawyers and risk managers: Patients do not sue people they like. Hopefully, you will never experience being called into a lawsuit, and if you think about how to get along with the patient and family/caregiver unit, you may avoid a lawsuit. Getting along with the patient and family/caregiver unit can be done in three steps:

1. Include the patient and family/caregiver unit in your plans for care.
2. Be observant, and do what is needed without having to be asked.
3. Do the little things that mean so much.

"The little things that mean so much" are the things that go beyond the expected. It is impossible to include all of these, but here is a partial list:

- Take a minute to talk with patients about their memories—wedding, children, job, special accomplishments.
- Use therapeutic touch. Touch their hand, arm, or back when talking with or greeting them.
- Change their bedspread for them.
- Take them a flower from your garden.
- Read a story to them—a chuckle for the day or a news event.
- Shave a woman's legs and underarms.
- Give patients a back rub and foot rub.
- Take a cassette tape of relaxing music for them to borrow.
- Discuss a movie you just saw.
- Take time to listen as they show you something special (grandchild's picture, mementos from vacations).
- Say "yes" to a cup of coffee or a glass of iced tea.

## THE DYING PATIENT

Everyone is going to die at some point in time. Not everyone has the gift of time that comes with a terminal illness. People diagnosed with terminal illnesses, such as

AIDS (acquired immune deficiency syndrome) or cancer, go through different emotions and thoughts. These were called the Stages of Grief by Dr. Elizabeth Kubler-Ross, a pioneer in the study of death and dying and a grief theorist.

## The Stages of Grief

### *Denial*

In this stage, patients do not believe that they have a terminal diagnosis. They think that it is a dream and they will wake up soon, or they think that the laboratory made a mistake. They decide that it does not feel like they are dying, and therefore, they are not dying. Some patients never leave this stage, possibly because denying their illness is the only way they can cope. To help patients through this stage:

- Listen to them.
- Be supportive.
- Be available and open to talk if they decide to talk.
- Let them take the lead.

### *Anger*

In this stage, patients realize that their diagnosis is terminal. They are dying, and they become angry. They wonder, "Why me?" Patients often take their anger out on those they love the most, their family. They may be unapproachable. They may throw things against the wall, yell at people, and make sarcastic comments to people trying to help. The best way to help patients through this stage is to:

- Be there for them.
- Listen quietly.
- Be supportive.
- Remain calm and do not get angry.

### Bargaining

During this stage, patients begin to bargain with a greater power (e.g., God, Buddha). They pray and make deals, such as if they are spared from this illness they will go to church every day or give money to charity. To help patients through this stage:

- Be supportive.
- Say, "That would be great if that happens."
- Listen without judgment.

### Depression

In this stage, patients allow themselves to recognize that they have a terminal illness and will be missing out on a lot of living. They become very sad about what they will never see and what they will miss. They may be very quiet. They may decide that they want to have control over their death and consider suicide. As a home care aide, you must be on the lookout for signs of depression and potential suicide. To help patients through this stage:

- Be supportive.
- Listen with empathy (put yourself in their place).
- Notify your supervisor and/or the patient's nurse.
- Try to talk about day-to-day activities.
- Tell them that you care and are available for them if they want to talk.

## *Acceptance*

This is the stage where the patient becomes peaceful and realistic. Many patients never reach this stage. If they do, you will watch them share a lot of love, feelings, and memories with those they love. During this stage you need to be supportive of the needs of the patient and family.

## Signs of Approaching Death

- The arms and legs become cold and turn bluish.
- The patient sleeps for longer periods of time.
- Respirations become very slow, deep, and long, and then periods without breathing occur.
- The patient stops eating and then stops drinking.
- The patient has difficulty swallowing saliva and therefore may drool.
- The patient becomes confused.

- The patient may pick at the sheets.
- The patient may lose control of feces and urine.
- The patient may see people and relatives who have died.

## CULTURAL AND ETHNIC DIFFERENCES

Sometimes health care providers jump to conclusions about patients and their families. Remember, just because they are not acting the way you would act in the same situation, do not assume that they are not normal. In reality their behavior may result from their culture or ethnic group. To learn more about your patients' cultural or ethnic background, you may want to ask them to explain some of their customs and beliefs. (Be aware of your nonverbal responses.) Some of the cultural differences include the following.

### Hispanic/Latino

- The family unit is strong:
  1. respect for elders first and foremost
  2. recognition of the role of the male as dominant.
- Beliefs about illness are based on religious beliefs (God's will).
- There is belief in the power of religious rites and icons to take away the illness.

- There is belief in the power of herbs to heal. Home remedy stores are available in most neighborhoods.
- People take care of their own families.
- The are very religious (usually Roman Catholic) and have religious icons throughout the home.
- Illness draws the entire family together.
- At the time of death, they cry so loudly that neighbors may hear.

## Asian

- Health is the result of free and positive energy flow.
- To have good health, there must be a balance between the negative forces (yin) and the positive forces (yang).
- Balance can be found through the use of herbs.
- There is belief in preventive practices such as
  1. meditation
  2. martial arts
  3. acumassage—massage done over the meridian points to rechannel the energy flow
  4. acupressure—pressure applied to the meridian points where energy flows
  5. moxibustion—a deep healing treatment in which a nine-year-old herb, moxa, is tied into a pellet and burned at an acupressure point until the patient feels the heat.

- When sick, cupping is done to draw out the bad energy. A bamboo cup is heated and put over the sick area of the skin. As the cup cools, it gets smaller and draws out the sickness.
- An alternative to cupping is pinching the sick area or applying deep pressure with a spoon. These practices produce bruises and can be mistaken for patient abuse.
- Public display of affection is avoided.

### African American

The beliefs of the African-American culture are based partly on the traditional health care beliefs from Africa, which include the following:

- Health can be influenced by the patient and family through knowledge and behavior.
- Singing and dancing brings the patient and family unit together.
- Illness is caused by bad spirits.
- Conjure men and women and voodoo doctors can get rid of bad spirits.
- Spiritual health is on the same plane as mental, physical, and emotional health.

African-American cultural characteristics include the following:

- They look to elders for guidance with what works.

- They use a combination of what the physician says, past experience, and trial and error.
- The extended family plays a role in health—brotherhood and sisterhood.
- Religious healing is possible.
- The elderly are to be respected and protected.
- They celebrate death with song and party.

## Native American

Although there are tribal variations, the following are attributed to all Native American cultures:

- They believe that handshakes are intrusive.
- They believe in the power of herbs and rituals of the medicine man.
- They place equal emphasis on the physical and the supernatural.
- They favor males.
- They support the extended family.
- They are ritualistic in grieving and burials.

## European

- Family-centered care is important.
- They will follow the physician's advice. The physician is revered as infallible.
- They are generally religious.
- They believe in folk remedies.

# CHAPTER 6

# Understanding Your Patient's Condition

## INTRODUCTION

Each patient has a diagnosis (a condition) or reason for needing home care. Because of this condition or need, a personal care provider (you) can be assigned to visit and care for the patient. Any time that you have a question about your assigned patient's condition, you should ask the nurse to whom you report about the patient's care. It is important that you know which signs and symptoms of the condition to report and what you might see because of the patient's condition. This can help you in your care as well as with concerns and needs of the patient and caregiver (person in the home with the patient).

## WHAT IT IS, WHAT IT MEANS, WHAT TO LOOK FOR, WHAT TO REPORT

The following sections address some of the common patient conditions that you will encounter. In each case, you need to know:

- what the condition is
- what the condition means
- what to look for
- what to report to the nurse
- what the patient needs because of the specific condition.

Anytime that you question anything the patient says or does, you can call the office and the nurse. When a patient or a caregiver has questions about the patient's condition or care, let the nurse know what the questions are so that he or she can answer them.

## Cerebral Vascular Accident (Stroke)

### *What Is It?*

This is a condition commonly seen in home care. It is commonly called a stroke. That means that the blood flow to the brain has been stopped for a period of time due to one of the following:

- a blood clot
- bleeding (hemorrhage)
- constricture (a spasm in the blood vessels)

A blood clot blocks the vessel so that blood with oxygen-carrying blood cells cannot get through. A hemorrhage means that a lot of blood is flowing, but it is not carrying the blood cells with oxygen to the brain. A spasm of the vessels causes the muscles to cramp and constrict. (It is similar to a leg cramp, only it happens in the blood vessels leading to the brain.)

### What Does It Mean?

This condition means that your patient has had some or all of the following signs and symptoms :

- weakness
- numbness
- slurred speech
- confusion
- disorientation
- difficulty with walking
- unsteady balance
- loss of bowel or bladder control
- headaches
- personality changes
- seeing problems, such as blurring of vision

Your patient has probably been in the hospital for this problem and has had an inpatient stay in a rehabilitation setting. The recovery from a stroke takes time. The care for a patient with a stroke depends on the symptoms that the patient has had.

## What Do You Look For?

You should look for a return or an increase in any of the signs and symptoms of a stroke listed above. The patient might also have side effects from medications. The patient is probably receiving a medication to make the blood thinner (an anticoagulant). This keeps the blood from forming clots. You should look for the following side effects of anticoagulant medication:

- blood in the urine or bowel movement
- bleeding of any kind
- gums that bleed and do not stop

Other signs and symptoms to look for are:

- increased fluid retention
- swelling of the legs and feet
- complaints by the patient of gaining weight

## What Do You Report?

If any return or increase in the signs and symptoms of a stroke occur while you are providing care or are reported to you by the patient or family/caregiver, you need to report this to the nurse. You also need to report any of the problems listed above that you see or that the patient and family/caregiver might tell you.

## Congestive Heart Failure

### *What Is It?*

This is a problem that occurs when the heart is not able to pump all the food and oxygen the body needs to all parts of the body. This can cause the blood to back up, like a clogged kitchen drain, and the backup is what causes the problems that patients have. Because of the slow movement of the blood or the backup of the blood, the body cannot get the oxygen and food it needs. The body is also unable to get rid of the bad wastes.

### *What Does It Mean?*

Patients with this problem have blood that backs up in the veins (the blood vessels that come back into the left side of the heart), and the blood continues to back up into the legs. Congestion in the legs leads to fluid, called edema. When the blood backs up from the right side of the heart, the fluid backs up into the lungs, and the patient will have breathing problems.

Patients with congestive heart failure are usually on a special diet. They are to limit the amount of salt in their diet because salt makes the body hold fluid, which in turn makes the heart have to pump harder, increasing the patient's symptoms. Do not use salt when you cook for the patient, and avoid foods such as

- lunch meats
- cheese

- pickles
- olives
- relish
- hot peppers
- canned soups
- canned meats
- frozen vegetables
- salty snacks such as chips, nuts, pretzels, and pop-corn

Encourage the patient to eat fresh vegetables and meats. Fruits are also a good thing to eat, whether they are canned, fresh, or frozen. Read the labels for the patient and the family/caregiver.

### What Do You Look For?

When you provide care for a patient with congestive heart failure (CHF), you will need to look for signs and symptoms of increasing backup of blood. What you see and what the patient complains about will depend on the side of the heart where the vessels are backing up the blood.

When the backup tends to be from the right side of the heart, look for

- shortness of breath
- fast breathing
- difficulty breathing when lying down
- difficulty breathing with activity
- cough

- fast heartbeat
- restlessness
- tiredness

When the backup is into the left side of the heart, the patient might complain of

- tight shoes
- swelling in the feet or ankles
- tight waistbands on clothes
- gaining weight
- getting up to urinate at night
- feeling tired
- tightness of rings

### *What Do You Report?*

It is important to report to the nurse any of the signs and symptoms listed above that you see or that the patient or family/caregiver complains about.

Whether you weigh the patient or the patient weighs him- or herself with help, remember to weigh

- at the same time of day
- in the same place
- with the same amount of clothes on each time
- on a flat, hard surface

Be sure to report to the nurse if:

- There is a weight gain of three pounds in any day.

- The patient's weight seems to be slowly going up each day.
- The patient is having problems getting the special food for his or her diet.

## Diabetes Mellitus (Sugar in the Blood)

### *What Is It?*

When the body (the pancreas, which is near the stomach) cannot give out insulin to break down the sugar that is eaten, the patient has diabetes or a sugar problem. Some patients need to take insulin, either by a needle injection or a pill, to replace what they do not have. This helps the patient's body use the food that is eaten by taking the food and breaking it apart into usable "fuel" for the body.

### *What Does It Mean?*

People who have family members with diabetes, who are very overweight, and who have a lot of stress over a long time are those who are likely to have diabetes. Sometimes women's bodies have a problem with using the food they eat when they are pregnant, and the woman appears to be diabetic. This type of diabetes (the kind that sometimes happens when a woman is pregnant) often goes away when the baby is born.

The diagnosis of diabetes can be either "non-insulin dependent," not needing to take in insulin by needle or pill, or "insulin dependent," needing to take in insulin in some form, usually by needle or pill. The patient will also be on a special diet. This diet is one that is limited in the amount of "sugar"-containing foods. The label of foods might say sucrose or fructose instead of sugar. It is important that you help the patient keep the diet. This means no sweets, but the patient can use saccharin or sweetener that does not contain sugar.

### What Do You Look For?

There are lots of signs and symptoms to look for in patients with the diagnosis of diabetes. It is important to know what they are.

*Low Blood Sugar.* If the patient is not getting enough food to keep the level of blood sugar high enough, the patient might complain of being hungry and dizzy. As you are providing care for the patient, you might notice that the patient is shakier or more irritable and nervous than usual. These symptoms might be a sign of a low blood sugar. Patients who have diabetes over a long time can often tell you how they feel and what to look for when caring for them. They might be tired and sweaty, and when they walk they might not be steady on their feet and seem to be lightheaded.

The nurse may have told you how important it is to give the patient something to eat when the patient complains of, or you see any sign of, low blood sugar. Give the patient:

- a piece of fruit **or**
- a piece or two of hard candy **or**
- some juice **or**
- soda **or**
- milk

Then call right away to tell the nurse what is happening. Remember to do the following:

- Talk with the nurse caring for the patient or another nurse in the office.
- Do not leave a message with the voice mail system unless you have also spoken with a nurse.
- Stay with the patient.
- See how the patient feels in about 10–15 minutes.
- Call back and tell the nurse how the patient feels.

*High Blood Sugar.* The signs that blood sugar is getting higher are much slower and occur over time. Patients might say that they are always thirsty or tired. They might also say they are sleeping a lot. They might seem to be uninterested in what is going on around them. When these things occur, it is important to tell the nurse about them. It is also important to encourage these patients to be as active as they are able to be and are allowed to be. If they are allowed to walk around the house, encourage them to walk with you beside them. It is also important to talk with patients about their diet. What has your patient been eating when you are not there? Who does his or her shopping and cooking? If the patient is able to answer these questions, you need to share the information with the nurse.

Skin care is very important in patients with diabetes. When you give or assist diabetic patients with a bath, be sure to look for open or dry and cracked areas on the skin. Try to keep the skin lubricated, especially in cold, wintry weather. You are not allowed to cut or file the nails of these patients. If they are becoming long, tell the nurse about it.

Some patients with diabetes wear a bracelet or necklace that says they are diabetic. If your patient has a bracelet or necklace that says this, be sure the patient wears it. If you take it off to give the patient a bath, be sure that you put it back on right away. It is important that the patient have this identification on at all times.

### What Do You Report?

- any signs and symptoms of low blood sugar:
  1. dizziness
  2. hunger
  3. shakiness
  4. nervousness
  5. irritability
  6. sweatiness

- 7. tiredness
- 8. sleepiness
- 9. unsteadiness
- any signs and symptoms of high blood sugar:
    1. thirst
    2. tiredness
    3. sleepiness
    4. lack of interest in what is going on around him or her
- skin that is cracked or dry
- nails that are long and need trimming
- problems with buying food
- eating things not allowed in the special diet
- poor appetite
- any signs and symptoms of a cold, such as
    1. stuffy head
    2. headaches
    3. fevers
    4. chills
    5. achy joints
- any signs and symptoms of stomach flu, such as
    1. nausea
    2. vomiting
    3. diarrhea

These are some of the things to look for and report to the nurse when you are assigned to care for a patient with diabetes. The nurse will tell you other things to look for and tell him or her about. But remember, if the patient has any sign of low blood sugar, give the patient what the nurse has told you to give and call the nurse!

## Myocardial Infarction (Heart Attack)

### What Is It?

A myocardial infarction is most often called an MI or a heart attack. It occurs when the blood supply to the heart muscle is blocked. The blood vessels (the part of the body that carries the blood) are small and become blocked because of fatty deposits, a clot of blood, or loss of the ability to be flexible (like a rubber band that stretches and shrinks when pulled and released). The blood cannot get through a vein or an artery, and part of the heart does not get what it needs to live. That part of the heart is said to have infarcted or "died," and new veins and arteries have to grow to take blood around the area and into the heart muscle. This is called new blood flow or circulation.

### What Does It Mean?

The patient must first rest the heart muscle and then begin to slowly increase activities over time as the physician orders. Followthrough with an after-heart-attack diet and medication plan is also important. The patient will usually have a special diet and medications pre-scribed by the physician. This plan includes a diet that

- is low in saturated fats (the fats that are solid at room temperature, such as lard)
- avoids high-sodium foods, such as pickles and pro-cessed cheese
- avoids salty snacks, such as chips and pretzels
- avoids canned soups, vegetables, and meats
- is low in caffeine (coffee and cola)
- is high in fresh vegetables
- is high in canned and fresh fruits
- is high in fish and poultry (skinned)
- is well balanced
- maintains but does not increase body weight
- is taken in small, frequent amounts

This patient will also probably have daily weights taken. You should remember that the patient must be weighed

- at the same time of day
- in the same place
- with same amount of clothes on each time
- on a flat, hard surface

Be sure to report to the nurse if:

- There is a weight gain of three pounds in any day.

- The patient's weight seems to be slowly going up each day.
- The patient's clothes or shoes are fitting too tightly.

It is important to assist this type of patient with dealing with stress and to provide a calm and relaxed setting for care. Your calm approach to assisting the patient with personal care and meal time preparation helps to keep the home relaxed and comfortable for the patient.

### *What Do You Look For?*

It is important to watch for the following signs and symptoms in heart attack patients:

- complaints of pain
- restlessness
- lots of sweating
- skin that is cool but moist to the touch
- increased weakness
- indigestion
- nausea and/or vomiting
- feelings of just not being "okay"
- weight gain
- clothes becoming too tight
- shoes becoming too tight
- foot or ankle swelling

Ask these patients about their diets. Do they know what they can eat and what they should not eat? Is there someone to pick up fresh foods at the grocery store and bring them home to prepare? How is their appetite?

If the patient is anxious, he or she might complain of stress. The patient probably wants someone to just listen. It is important not to share your personal problems with the patient and family/caregiver but rather to be a good listener.

### *What Do You Report?*

When you provide care to a patient who has had a heart attack, be sure to report the changes in weight or appetite and any signs and symptoms the patient has (see the lists above). It is also important to let the nurse know about the patient and family/caregiver's concerns regarding:

- stress
- meal preparation
- availability of food
- anxiety
- nervousness
- anything else unusual for the patient

If the patient seems to be overly tired rather than having more energy over a period of time, it is also important to report this back to the nurse.

### The Dying Patient

Whether the agency you work for is a hospice or a home health agency, you will most likely find yourself caring for patients whose life expectancy is limited due to a specific illness or condition or due to the aging process. Many individuals cared for by home health agencies are very elderly and frail.

### What Is It?

Any patient who has a progressively worsening illness or who is not expected to live beyond six months can be considered a dying patient. Some of the more common diagnoses of patients who are considered to be dying are

- AIDS (acquired immune deficiency syndrome)
- CHF (congestive heart failure)
- cancer

### What Does It Mean?

Dying patients and their families/caregivers need lots of emotional support and kindness in the provision of care. It is important to ask the nurse if the patient and/or family/caregiver know that the patient is dying. This is not something you should discuss with the patient or family/caregiver unless you know that they know the seriousness of the patient's condition.

If the nurse does not tell you, be sure to ask if the patient wants to be resuscitated if he or she stops breathing. If you are trained in cardiopulmonary resuscitation (CPR), then you should have the necessary equipment (airway) to provide CPR safely. You should also know the wishes of your patients and their family/caregivers in this regard. If they do not want CPR, then they must put their wishes into writing and the physician must sign an order to this effect. It is important to know this about all your patients, not just those who are actively dying.

It is also important to know if patients have pain and, if they do, what you, as an aide, can do to help relieve the patient's pain. Things that you might be able to do to decrease a patient's pain are

- positioning the patient in a specific position of comfort
- providing a back rub to the patient
- reading to take the patient's mind off of the pain
- offering the patient frequent fluids
- providing good skin care
- toileting the patient frequently
- rubbing his or her forehead

### *What Do You Look For?*

With dying patients or family/caregivers of patients who are dying, there are some important things to look for during care:

- decreased output (urine)
- constipation
- diarrhea

- decreased appetite
- extreme sleepiness
- inability to sleep
- increased pain
- talking about suicide
- the patient's lack of interest in what is happening around him or her
- fatigue on the part of the family/caregiver

These patients require lots of good personal care, as well as a kind and caring caregiver. Take time with patients and their family/caregivers and listen to their concerns. Give them a chance to talk about their feelings, but most importantly, remember to listen and to be supportive. Making these patients comfortable and keeping them clean and dry is very important.

### *What Do You Report?*

It is important to report any of the signs and symptoms listed above to the nurse. If the family/caregiver is becoming overly tired from caring for the patient, the nurse might be able to arrange for someone to provide respite care. This could mean having someone stay in the home overnight so that the family/caregiver can get a full night's rest and sleep. It can also mean providing someone during the day for several hours so that the family/caregiver can go out for a few hours.

If the patient speaks about suicide, it is important to report this back to the nurse. A social worker or someone skilled in counseling patients can come to the home to talk with the patient and family/caregiver.

If you have been asked to take the patient's vital signs (i.e., pulse, respirations, temperature, and blood pressure), be certain to do so and report any changes to the nurse. The nurse will tell you specific levels of pulse, respirations, temperature, and blood pressure that should be reported for individual patients.

## Chronic Obstructive Pulmonary Disease (Congested Lungs)

This condition causes breathing problems and occurs over a long time. There are two types of chronic obstructive pulmonary disease (COPD), and it is important to know which one your patient has been diagnosed as having. Both conditions mean that the patient has difficulty breathing out the air taken in.

### *What Is It?*

Sometimes workers in plants where there is a lot of asbestos or air pollution will come down with COPD in later years. Often they will have problems with colds and breathing when they are younger. Many times these patients did not realize that it was related to work or smoking, another cause of COPD in later years.

The first type of COPD is also called emphysema. This means that the small air sacs (like little balloons) within the lungs become stiff, like an old rubber band. They might dry out and break open, or they might not be able to push the air back out, resulting in air being trapped in the lungs.

The second type of COPD might also be called chronic bronchitis. This is when the bronchioles (tubes into the lungs) have lots of secretions. These secretions can be lots of really thick sputum or infected sputum that can become pus. All of the secretions build up and block the flow of air. In this case, even the membranes (the covering of the lungs) are thickened, and breathing becomes more and more difficult, with more and more air being trapped in the lungs.

### *What Does It Mean?*

Patients with the diagnosis of COPD should be watched for signs and symptoms of emphysema and chronic bronchitis. They are similar and you will not need to know the difference in symptoms for reporting, just what you need to look for. The patient with chronic bronchitis might have frequent cold symptoms.

Both of these conditions mean that the patient needs

- to have lots of rest
- to have lots of fluids

- to have small frequent feedings in small quantities
- to avoid drafts
- to avoid individuals with colds
- to eat a well-balanced diet

Patients with COPD might find it easier to breathe in certain positions. It is important to know what these positions are for the individual patient. Some examples of positions and techniques that might make it easier for the patient with COPD to breath are

- sitting upright
- leaning forward over a stand
- pursing lips (like getting ready to kiss someone) while breathing
- breathing in and holding, then releasing the air back out

When patients with COPD become upset and anxious, their breathing is more difficult. Help the patient to relax and be calm. You should provide good personal care with a calm and confident approach and listen to the patient if he or she is upset or anxious.

Remember to use good universal precautions (i.e., gloves and masks) when caring for these patients and to provide tissues and a plastic bag close by the patient for disposing of used tissues. Good handwashing technique is important for you, the patient, and the family/caregiver.

## *What Do You Look For?*

If your patient has emphysema, look for

- increasing breathing problems with movement
- cough, which is usually dry

If your patient has more of a problem with chronic bronchitis, look for

- shortness of breath
- respirations that sound wheezy
- a lot of sputum when coughing, especially in the morning
- signs and symptoms of an infection, such as elevated temperature and cold symptoms

## *What Do You Report?*

As with any patient, be certain to report any patient complaints or changes in the patient. It is especially important to report any of the above symptoms, as well as any

- temperature elevation above 101° by mouth
- increasingly difficult breathing
- increase in amount of sputum
- changes in the color of the sputum; bloody, rusty, greenish sputum
- poor appetite
- decreased respirations

Besides looking for the signs and symptoms to report, it is also important to report other things to the nurse. These include how the patient is feeling. For example, is the patient anxious or calm? Is the patient taking his or her medicines? Does the patient continue to smoke? Is the patient able to provide any or all self-care without becoming exhausted and being unable to breathe?

Patients with COPD might be receiving oxygen. If so, please refer to Chapter 8 for guidelines in caring for the patient who is receiving oxygen.

## The Total Hip Patient (Hip Fractures and Replacements)

In a total hip replacement, the head of the femur, the long bone in the top part of the leg, is replaced. This means that the patient will be limited in mobility for a time and will be in need of your care while the bone heals.

### *What Is It?*

A total hip replacement occurs for one of several reasons. The first is because the bone is no longer strong. This happens as people age because bones become more porous, like Swiss cheese. The hip needs to be replaced because of an ongoing process in which there is decreased bone strength and joints become more difficult to move. Joints might also be painful and stiff.

Another reason for a total hip replacement is a broken hip. The hip might have broken because the patient is elderly and the bones are not strong. The hip might also have broken because of a cancer that gets into the bones and makes them brittle and easily broken.

Other patients will fall or be injured (e.g., in an automobile accident) and have a broken hip. In some cases it is not necessary to do a total hip replacement. Instead, the broken hip is put back into place and kept in place while healing occurs. But most often in home care, patients with broken hips have a total hip replacement.

### *What Does It Mean?*

There will probably be a physical therapist involved in patient care, and you might be asked to provide some range of motion exercises as part of your care. It is important to understand what exercise the patient is allowed and to follow the plan of care exactly. If the patient tells you he or she is able to do more or did do more over the weekend when you were not providing care, clarify this with the nurse or physical therapist. Ask what the patient can do before changing your personal care routine.

Hip replacement patients will have an incision (cut) from surgery. The dressing will be changed by the nurse or family/caregiver, once the family/caregiver has been taught to change the dressing. If the family/caregiver is changing the dressing and tells you about the incision, make certain you share this information with the nurse.

The patient will have to gradually increase both the amount of weight put on the hip and the amount of walking he or she can do. The patient might start off walking with a walker and progress to a cane during the period when you are providing personal care. The patient will need to use helping equipment (walker, cane, etc.) as directed and with all mobility.

The patient also needs to follow some activity suggestions, including these:

- Dress starting with the affected side.
- Use adaptive dressing equipment for reaching and self-care.
- Avoid rushing to do tasks.
- Sit when possible to do tasks to save energy.
- Store items in the kitchen and bathroom within easy reach (Gingerich & Ondeck, 1997).

When you provide care to patients with a total hip replacement, it is important that you assist them in following the suggestions above. Ask patients what they use most often in the kitchen and whether you can put these items down lower, perhaps on the countertop. Reassure the patient and family/caregiver that the movement of these items is temporary. After the hip has healed and mobility is back to normal, you will help them move the items back to the cabinet. Do the same thing for the patient and family/caregiver in the bathroom and the bedroom.

### What Do You Look For?

With the patient who has had a total hip replacement, no matter what the reason, the following are important things to look for and to do:

- Watch to be certain that the patient is using his helping equipment (e.g., walker, cane, etc.).
- Make certain the patient is not sitting with the sore leg over the other leg.
- Keep the sore hip in no more than a 90° angle when the patient is sitting straight up.
- Keep the hip from turning inward.
- Make certain that throw rugs are put away.
- Keep the patient's pathways free of clutter.
- Assist the patient with personal care and meal preparation.
- Remind the patient to conserve (not use up) his or her energy.
- Remind the patient of exercises and assist with them when they are ordered.
- Ask the patient if he or she has pain.
- Take the patient's temperature if directed to do so.

### What Do You Report?

Report to the nurse if the patient or family/caregiver tells you any of the following about the incision:

- The incision is warm.
- The incision is red.

- There is drainage.
- There is pain or tenderness.

It is also important to let the nurse know if the patient:

- has a temperature over 101°F by mouth
- has pain
- has increased difficulty with using the helping equipment
- has difficulty understanding the exercise program
- does not want to follow the activity restrictions
- has questions about his or her care

## CONCLUSION

Patients that you care for within the home care setting have many conditions. Those discussed here are some of the more common conditions of patients cared for by home care aides. It is important that you understand the patient's condition so that you are able to provide the best of care. When you are assigned a new patient whose condition is not one of those listed above, ask the nurse to tell you the following:

- What is this condition?
- What does this condition mean?
- What should I look for?
- What do you want me to report about this patient?
- Are there any special needs of this patient and family/caregiver?

You could also ask the nurse to give you a copy of the information used for patient teaching about the condition and signs and symptoms so that you could add this information to your pocket guide. You might find that the pocket guide is not big enough for the information. A binder with dividers would be a good way to organize the information. With more complete information about your patients' conditions, the personal care you provide becomes even better. Your patients and their family/caregivers are pleased with your care and you feel a sense of satisfaction about your work.

Most importantly, remember to ask questions when you are unsure. Report back to the nurse when asked to look for signs and symptoms and report, as well as when you observe anything different about the patient and family/caregiver while providing care in the home.

Finally, remember that all information about your patients is confidential. Any information that has a patient's name or address on it should not be shared with anyone and should be returned to be destroyed in the home care office.

# CHAPTER 7

# Your Personal Safety

## INTRODUCTION

Safety in the provision of home care is very important. Chapter 6 discussed patient safety:

- what to look for
- what to do
- what to report
- what to ask the patient and family/caregiver
- what the patient's condition means in terms of providing safe care

Now it is time to think about your safety while providing care in the home setting. Your safety while providing care is very important. It is just as important as the patient's and/or family/caregiver's safety. Following the suggestions and guidelines in this manual will help to keep you safer when providing care as a home care aide.

This chapter is divided into sections that address:

- patient-related safety
- environmental safety
- prevention

Each of these areas is equally important to your safety. If you have any questions about the information provided, please ask your home care aide supervisor. It is important that you understand how these areas of safety affect your well-being.

## PATIENT-RELATED SAFETY

You are assigned to care for many different patients. When you go from one home to another, it is important that you do not carry germs from one patient to another. It is also important that you do not carry germs to yourself or to your family. In addition, as a home care aide, you are asked to provide a variety of personal care services to your patients, including lifting, transferring, and moving patients. This means you need to use proper precautions in the movement of patients in order to protect yourself. For your health and safety, you need to understand areas of patient safety.

## Handling Patient Wastes

Patient wastes come in many different forms, including any kind of secretion or drainage that comes from a patient. When you provide personal care for patients, you come in contact with drainage such as

- feces (bowel movements)
- urine
- saliva or sputum
- nasal secretions
- sinus drainage (from the eyes, nose, or throat)
- blood from cuts or bruises
- vomitus from upset stomachs
- vaginal and seminal fluids
- any fluid or droplets that come from the patient

You therefore must protect

- yourself from the patient's germs
- your patient from other patient's germs
- your patient from his or her own germs

The best thing to do to keep germs from spreading is to use good handwashing technique. Your agency probably has a policy on handwashing. You must follow your agency's policy, but if the agency has no policy, follow these steps:

1. Use liquid antibacterial soap.
2. Place the soap on a protective barrier in the home; that is, place a paper towel between the bottle of soap and whatever you set it on in the home.
3. Turn on the water.
4. Make certain the water is very warm to hot. Do not use cold water.
5. Wet hands.
6. Squeeze several drops of liquid soap on your hands.
7. Lather hands well.
8. Briskly rub hands under the running hot water.
9. Rinse the soap off your hands.
10. Use another paper towel to turn off the water.
11. Use another paper towel to dry your hands.
12. Discard the paper towel.
13. Replace soap into your bag.
14. Close your bag.

Once your hands are clean, you should use the protective supplies the agency provides. Use gloves when providing care of any kind. Use an apron (plastic) when providing a bath in bed or in a shower or anytime that your uniform might become damp. Wear a mask if the patient has a respiratory infection or if you think you might be splashed by the patient's secretions. In addition to a mask over your mouth and nose, you might also need to wear plastic protective goggles over your eyes or over your glasses.

### Transporting Patient Wastes

It is not a good idea to transport any patient wastes. You should never transport patient wastes unless the organization tells you it is okay. If you are asked to do this by the organization, be sure to follow these basic rules:

- Keep the wastes in a confined area in your vehicle (car).
- Keep them inside a closed container.
- Keep the lid of the container on tightly.
- Double-bag the wastes before removing them from the patient's home.
- Label the container "Patient Waste."

## Back Safety

### Body Mechanics: Position and Technique

The practice of good body mechanics is important to your health and safety. Good body mechanics means that you use your body effectively, with good posture and position. Patients are heavy, and moving and lifting patients can be tiring on muscles and limbs. Here are some hints for keeping your back and body healthy:

- Keep your back in good posture to decrease fatigue.
- Stand with your back straight and hips tucked in.
- Keep your shoulders straight.
- Keep your head erect.
- Keep your weight spread over your bottom, your hips, and your thighs.

### Lifting and Moving

When lifting, it is important to maintain a wide base of support. That means keeping your feet about 12 inches apart. Bring the patient or object to be lifted close to your body, and follow these steps:

1. Keep back straight.
2. Stoop to a squatting position.
3. Keep objects to be lifted close to your body.
4. Lift with legs and thighs by straightening legs.
5. Tighten stomach and bottom muscles.
6. Rise to a standing position.

Some other important rules in moving items from one spot to another are the following:

- Do not twist.
- Do not turn.
- Use a pivot technique.
- Keep your feet facing the direction of the pull or lift.
- Use a back support.

- Keep the lifted item's weight evenly distributed.
- Maintain your balance at all times.

### *Transferring Patients*

Patient transfers include moving patients from bed to chair, chair to bed, chair to toilet, chair to tub, and many others. Transfers also include moving patients up in the bed or to a sitting position. It is good to learn the best way to do transfers. Many times patients are bigger than you are, and proper transferring is important to both your safety and the patient's safety. If a therapist (physical or occupational) is providing care to the patient, he or she can assist you in understanding the best and easiest way to accomplish the transfer or movement desired.

*Moving the Patient Up in Bed.*
1. Put down side rail on the side of bed where you are standing.
2. Place the arm closest to the patient under the patient's arm.
3. Stand close to the bed.
4. Move your arm up under the patient's shoulder.
5. Place your other arm under the patient's head and shoulder.
6. Have patient bend legs at knees.
7. Establish a signal.
8. Ask patient to push upward with feet at the signal.

9. As patient pushes, lift up patient's head and shoulders slightly and pull patient toward the top of the bed.
10. Reposition patient comfortably.
11. Raise bed side rail, if present.

*Transferring Patient from Bed to Chair.* It is always important to have everything ready for the patient's transfer before you begin. If you are moving the patient out of bed and into a chair, these are the steps to follow:

1. Get the chair and place it by the bed.
2. Lock the wheels if the chair is a wheelchair.
3. Have the patient's robe (if needed) on the chair.
4. Lock arms with the patient to move the patient to a sitting position.
5. Rotate hips of patient so that patient is sitting on the edge of the bed with legs dangling.
6. Stand in front of the patient.
7. Put the robe on the patient.
8. Keep your feet about 12 inches apart.
9. Keep your knees bent.
10. Keep your feet by both feet of the patient to secure their placement.
11. Place patient's hands on your shoulders.
12. Put your hands under the patient's arms.
13. Bend knees.

14. On a prearranged count (e.g., 1, 2, 3), support and stand and pivot patient.
15. Make sure the backs of the patient's legs are against the chair seat.
16. Lower patient into chair.

The above directions for moving a patient can be used when lifting anything. Remember to protect your back and yourself when lifting. Many organizations now provide back supports for their employees to wear when lifting. These should fit snugly and be worn correctly so that they can do the job they are designed to do. Protect your back! Anytime you are unclear about the best way to lift a patient, remember to ask the nurse or physical therapist to show you.

**Infection Control**

You need to prevent infections to yourself and to your patients. Most organizations provide staff with lots of protective equipment. Items you need to prevent infections include

- liquid soap and towels (for handwashing)
- waterless hand cleaner for homes without running water (for handwashing)
- equipment bag (to be protected from contact with the home by setting it on a hard surface covered by a newspaper or paper towels)

- latex gloves (worn when coming in contact with blood or body fluids)
- plastic aprons (worn when splashing or soiling from blood or body fluids might occur)
- masks (worn when patients or family/caregivers are actively coughing)
- masks (worn when you have an upper respiratory infection with coughing and/or very runny nose)
- goggles (worn when splashing of blood or body fluids might occur)
- antireflux respirator (used when providing cardiopulmonary resuscitation)
- face shields (to be taken with you and used with ventilator patients)

When the equipment you have been given is not disposable, you need to clean it the way the organization directs you to clean it. Most organizations still use either an alcohol or a disinfectant wipe. The wipe is used to wipe off equipment after use and then is placed in a plastic bag to be returned to the agency for better cleaning prior to being returned to the bag. But what else should you be doing? If the item is something you need to use again, such as a blood pressure cuff, follow these guidelines:

- Protect the cuff with plastic wrap (when your patient has any known infectious disease).

- Still wipe the blood pressure cuff with alcohol or a disinfectant wipe or spray.
- Do not take your bag or equipment into homes where there is a lot of drainage and patient germs.
- Remember to also keep separate areas of your car for 'clean' and 'unclean' supplies.
- Keep handwashing supplies in an outside part of your bag.
- When in doubt, wash your hands again.

When the organization offers a review of infection control practices, be sure to attend. It is very important to you, your family, and your patients that you know what you need to do to prevent the spread of germs.

## Universal Precautions

You hear the words "universal precautions" often in any health care setting. These words mean that it is important to consider everyone and everything as a potential source of infection. You need to use protective items, such as gloves, with everyone. Even if you think there are no germs present, wear the appropriate protective gear, such as gloves, and wash your hands. Germs cannot be seen, and many times germs are present long before a patient has any sign of an illness. Be safe and be prepared. Use universal precautions all of the time.

## ENVIRONMENTAL SAFETY*

Home care aides work in a variety of settings and are exposed to a range of situations, for example:

- transportation settings—automobile, public transportation
- travel settings—roads, sidewalks
- onsite settings (patient care settings)—homes, apartment buildings, personal care homes

These categories fit into several areas of safety. They are transportation safety, travel safety, and patient care environment safety.

### Transportation Safety

#### *Automobile*

Your car should be kept in good working order. There are a number of preventive things you can do to maintain your car:

- Take it in for routine maintenance checks.
- Replace worn belts.
- Replace tires with poor tread.

---

*Source: Reprinted with permission from *The Home Health Aide Educator,* 1998, ADVANTAGE Health Care Management Resources Press.

- Keep the spare tire inflated.
- Check the oil, water, and brake fluid levels at regular intervals.
- Fill the gasoline tank when it is half empty.
- Keep the windshield washer fluid tank filled.
- Replace worn windshield wipers.

In addition, always wear your seatbelt for safety.

## *Public Transportation (Bus, Cab, Trolley, Train)*

Safe, reliable transportation is very important to your job and your safety. In addition to traveling by car, you might also need to use public transportation (bus, cab, trolley, or commuter train) to get to and from your patient's home. Here are some tips on the safe use of public transportation:

- Do not get into public transportation when there are individuals who appear suspicious.
- Use well-lighted transportation stops.
- Choose a seat close to the driver.
- Do not wait at a transportation stop alone.
- Observe who gets off at your stops.
- Do not get off at a stop where you do not feel safe.
- Do not talk to strangers.
- Do not tell strangers where you are going.

## Travel Safety

Safe traveling includes driving, walking, and using streets and roadways.

## *Driving*

It is important to be aware of the following safe driving practices:

- Obey all traffic laws.
- Keep money on hand for road emergencies when you might need to take a cab.
- Know ahead of time where you are going.
- Plan the safest route to get to your destination.
- Know the location of public buildings that are open and staffed 24 hours a day, such as police stations.
- If you think that someone is following you, drive to the nearest police station.
- Do not stop along a deserted road for any reason.
- Park in well-lighted areas.
- Do not pick up hitchhikers.
- Do not offer rides to strangers or family/caregivers.
- Keep valuables, such as your purse, out of sight.
- Wear your seatbelt when the car is moving.
- Lock your car doors while driving or parking.
- Take the car keys with you when leaving the car.

## *Roads*

You should be prepared to handle vehicle breakdowns in the following situations:

- On a major highway:
  1. Stay with the car.
  2. Transfer to the passenger seat to give the impression that you are not traveling alone.
  3. Only open the window a few inches to ask any "good Samaritans" to call the police for help.
- In a well-known or active area:
  1. Place a white piece of cloth out the driver's side window.
  2. Walk briskly to a pay phone or the home of an acquaintance.
- In winter:
  1. Make sure the tailpipe is unobstructed before idling the car.
  2. Turn the car off when the chill is gone from the car.
  3. Alternate idling the car for warmth and turning the car off to preserve fuel.
  4. Stay warm by wrapping yourself in emergency blankets and clothes. (Carry these in your car at all times.)
  5. Stay dry by using the emergency clothes.

When returning home:

- Scan the area around the garage or parking area.
- Drive on if you see suspicious persons.
- Go to a safe place, such as a police station.

*Walkways*

When you are returning to your car:

- Have the key out to unlock the car.
- Do not fumble with the lock.
- Keep keys firmly between the fingers of your dominant hand so that they are not dropped if you are bumped from behind.

When using walkways, follow these guidelines:

- Walk with a purpose.
- Look forward.
- Scan the area into which you are walking.
- Do not walk into loitering groups.
- Be alert for noises behind you and at your sides.
- Do not become preoccupied.
- Do not carry your purse. If you must carry a purse, keep it out of sight or held closely against your body.
- Follow known pathways when possible.
- Do not walk between buildings.
- Avoid deserted areas.
- Avoid alleys.
- Avoid poorly lit areas.
- Never accept a ride from anyone you do not know.
- Carry and use a repellent spray, if necessary.

When returning home, follow these suggestions in addition to those above:

- If driven, ask driver to wait until you are inside.
- Have your key out.
- Keep the key firmly in your hand.
- Do not enter your home if something appears unusual; instead, return to the vehicle and drive to the nearest police station.

## Patient Care Environment Safety

### *General Rules*

- Do not enter any location if you observe suspicious activity outside.
- Go to the nearest pay phone in a safe location.
- Call your supervisor for instructions.
- Ask your supervisor about escort services for high-risk areas.
- Do not proceed if in doubt.
- Inform the office of any abnormal occurrence.
- Do not wear expensive jewelry or clothing.
- Do not carry large amounts of money.
- Dress appropriately in conservative clothing.
- Do not enter any patient care setting where abuse of controlled substances is suspected.
- Do not give out any information to unknown persons on the telephone.

### *Homes*

- Confirm the address before entering.
- Ask permission to come into the home.
- Ask the person answering the door whose home it is.
- Determine who is present in the home upon entering.
- Be aware of others' location in the home.
- Look for alternative exits (doors or windows) from the home.
- Look to see who is at the door prior to opening the door.
- Call out to another person to indicate that you are not alone when going to the door.
- Keep chain locks in place when answering the door.
- Ask for identification from anyone who comes to the door.
- Do not allow strangers in to make telephone calls. Instead, offer to make a call while the stranger waits outside.
- If threatening behavior occurs within the home, excuse yourself and go to the nearest secure pay phone to report behavior. Then do not reenter the home.
- Keep yourself between individuals and exits if you have concerns.
- Do not allow those with questionable motives to come between you and the exit.

- If threatened, leave your patient care supplies and consider your safety as the primary concern.

## *Apartment Buildings*

- Do not allow strangers in the security door of the apartment building.
- Be observant.
- Confirm the location of the apartment.
- Do not get into elevators with suspicious individuals.
- Avoid dark stairwells unless accompanied by an escort or another person.
- Report any burnt-out hall lights.
- Call and have a family member or friend of the patient meet you at the entrance.
- Confirm who is present in the apartment prior to entering.
- Be aware of others' location in the apartment.
- Once inside the apartment, follow the same rules as listed for homes.
- If threatening behavior occurs within the apartment, excuse yourself and go to the nearest secure pay phone to report behavior. Then do not reenter the apartment.
- Keep yourself between individuals and exits if you have concerns.
- Do not allow those with questionable motives to come between you and the exit.

- If threatened, leave your patient care supplies and consider your safety as the primary concern.

### *Personal Care Homes*

- Confirm the identification of your patient.
- Determine others present in the personal care home.
- Be aware of others' location in the personal care home.
- Avoid dark stairwells unless accompanied by an escort or another person.
- Call and have a family member or friend of the patient meet you at the entrance.
- Once inside the personal care home, follow the same rules as listed for homes.
- If threatening behavior occurs within the personal care home, excuse yourself and go to the nearest secure pay phone to report behavior. Then do not re-enter the personal care home.
- Keep yourself between individuals and exits if you have concerns.
- Do not allow those with questionable motives to come between you and the exit.
- If threatened, leave your patient care supplies and consider your safety as the primary concern.

## Pet Safety

When providing care for patients, it is important to be relaxed around any pets that might be in the patient's home setting. However, remember that you are a stranger to the pet. You never know how a pet might react to your presence within the home setting. The following are some good rules to follow with pets or animals discovered while providing care for home care patients:

- Never approach an animal you do not know.
- If the patient's pet(s) is making you uncomfortable, ask the patient or family/caregiver to put the pet into another room.
- Inform your supervisor of any pet allergies you have.
- If pets are allowed to move about the house freely, ask for the pet to be placed in a cage or a separate room prior to your arrival.
- Call ahead and let the patient or family/caregiver know when you are arriving so that the pet can be secured.
- Do not hold pets, because pet hair might cause an allergic reaction in your other patients.

- Remember to wash your hands completely after any contact with an animal, bird, or other pet.
- Remind the patient and family/caregiver to keep the patient care area clean and free from pet waste.
- Remind the patient and family/caregiver to keep medications out of reach of any pets.
- Remind the patient and family/caregiver to keep any patient wastes out of reach of any pets.

**Fire Safety**

Fire in the home can be a major threat, especially to the elderly population. Your patients are in constant danger of a home fire. There are many important fire prevention clues to look for when caring for a patient in the home setting. Since one of the most common causes for fires is electrical wiring, look for the following things, and tell the patient, family/caregiver, and nurse if you spot them:

- frayed electrical cords
- too many plugs in an outlet
- sparks from any outlet
- electric cords under carpet
- three-prong adapters that are not grounded
- patient or family/caregiver using electric appliances near the sink or tub
- any exposed wires
- wires that are taped together

- bulbs of high wattage in outlets that specify low-wattage bulbs only

Smoking in bed is another major reason for home fires. To help prevent fires started by smoking:

- Remind the patient not to smoke in bed.
- Put out lit cigarettes or cigars, and throw out smoking tobacco into a large, heavy ashtray.
- Empty ashtrays when only partly full.
- Make sure ashes are cool before discarding.
- Discard ashes into sand, water, or a metal container.
- Do not allow patients on oxygen to smoke.
- Make certain that the "no smoking" sign stays posted.
- Remind visitors and family/caregivers not to smoke around oxygen.
- Keep matches in a safe place.
- Keep wool and synthetic items away from oxygen units.

You should also remember, and remind your patients and family/caregivers, of other important home fire safety hints, including these:

- Close the bedroom door when asleep, because a door slows fire down.
- Do not let trash cans overflow.
- Do not keep old paper and newspapers.
- Do not leave the stove on if no one is in the kitchen.

- Keep the top of stoves and heat vents clear.
- Do not place items on top of heaters.

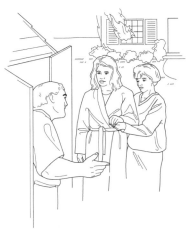

If a fire should start in a home when you are present, it is important to have planned ahead. Know at least two different ways to get out of the home. Know the fire emergency numbers. In the event of a fire, use the safest (furthest) exit. Plan, in advance, to meet the patient and family/caregiver at a safe place outside. If there is someone in the family who can help you get the patient safely out of the home, use his or her help. Know ahead of time if any of the windows are locked or painted shut and cannot be opened. Remember to remain calm at the time of a fire or any other problem and to follow these guidelines:

- In an apartment building, feel doors for heat before opening them.
- Do not open a hot door.
- If the exits are blocked by fire, place wet towels at the bottom of any doors.
- Keep the smoke out of the room.
- If time permits, cover your face and the patient's face with a damp cloth.

- Leave the burning area (home).
- Close doors behind you to keep the door between you and the fire.
- If it is safe to do so, first vacate and then call in the fire from a phone in a safe location (a neighbor's phone).
- Make certain the patient and family/caregivers are safe.
- Call the office to report:
  1. what has happened
  2. who is with you
  3. where you are
  4. how you can be reached
- Follow the directions given to you by the agency.
- Do not leave the patient until someone (family/caregiver) is present or you are directed to do so by the home health agency staff.
- If you are moved from the location reported to the agency (by firefighters, ambulance, or other means), call again to report your location.
- Remember to have a plan and to follow it.

### *Fire Extinguishers and Smoke Detectors*

- Know what types of fire extinguishers are present within the home setting.
- Make certain that the extinguishers are in working condition.
- Know the location of any smoke detectors or fire extinguishers present within the home setting.

- Ask your patient or family/caregiver when smoke detectors were last checked.
- Tell the nurse what information the patient and family/caregiver give you about any fire extinguishers or smoke detectors.
- Ask the nurse to explain:
  1. how to use any fire extinguishers present
  2. the best exit route from the home care setting
  3. how to best move the patient

### *Fire Alarms*

In personal care homes and apartment house settings, fire alarms are present. Locate the fire alarms when assigned to patients in these care settings. If you smell smoke or suspect a fire is present, and if time allows, pull the alarm and vacate the building. Never take time to pull the alarm when you and/or the patient are in danger.

## PREVENTION

### Preemployment Screening

Employee health is important to the home care agency. At the time of employment, most organizations will ask you to have a recent physical examination and a complete health history by a physician approved by the organization. In addition to the history and physical, the following tests are usually conducted:

- a routine urinalysis
- a complete blood count
- two negative tuberculosis tests
- a negative chest X-ray, if indicated (if there is a positive tuberculosis test)

## Immunizations

Most home care agencies will conduct an immunization history when you are hired. Some immunizations (which protect you from illnesses) are offered or recommended to you by the home care agency. Tests that help to tell whether you need immunizations or not include

- a rubeola titer (if your birthdate is after 1956)
- a rubella titer

Some home care agencies also offer staff who have negative results from these tests vaccines for rubeola and rubella. The home care agency also gives staff three injections (shots) of hepatitis B vaccine. These are offered within 10 days of employment to all employees who have a potential for blood and/or body fluid exposure.

Ask for information about immunizations and specifically about hepatitis B. Education about immunizations is important so that you understand what to look for and what having the shots means. If you are a woman, ask what any immunization means if you are pregnant. Once you have been taught about the hepatitis B series of shots, you can refuse the series. If you have had these immunizations before, do not repeat the series unless you did not complete all three shots. For you to be immunized, it is important that you have all three shots in the series and that they are spaced the right amount of time apart. If you decide to refuse the series you must sign a special form.

## Ongoing Testing

Staff who are assigned to care for patients who have tuberculosis (TB) or patients at high risk of getting tuberculosis, such as alcoholics, prisoners, and patients who are HIV (human immunodeficiency virus) positive, will usually be given a Mantoux test (TB test) every six months. For other at-risk staff, this test is done only once a year. Sometimes if staff have signs and symptoms that resemble tuberculosis, the home health agency will ask them to have another Mantoux test. It is a good idea to have the test so that if you are ill you can get medicines and be treated.

Some organizations also offer staff the influenza (flu) vaccine. It is your decision whether to have a flu vaccine or not. Ask for information about the vaccine and the flu before you decide what you want to do.

## Healthy Practices

The home health organization wants to keep you healthy. If you should develop an illness, most agencies have guidelines regarding reporting to work, for example:

- Call your supervisor to report off work if you have a temperatuve of 101°F or higher.
- Tell the supervisor your symptoms to be recorded in the employee illness log.
- Tell the scheduler when you have a cold (without a fever).
- Report any symptoms of gastrointestinal upset (nausea, vomiting, and diarrhea) to the office.
- Report any communicable diseases that your children or family members have, such as measles, mumps, or chicken pox.

Often part of the organization's performance improvement is tracking employee illnesses. By letting the organization know when you are ill, you help improve the organization and patient care.

## CONCLUSION

Protect yourself and protect others. Use the suggestions provided to keep yourself and your patients safe. If you do not understand or do not remember something you have been told, always ask for direction. You are important to the organization and your patients, and the agency wants you to be safe and secure.

# CHAPTER 8

# Correct Equipment Use

As a home care aide, you will need to use different types of mechanical aids to care for patients. It is important that you understand not only how to use the equipment in a safe manner but also what you can and cannot accept responsibility for while using the equipment.

## PATIENT CARE EQUIPMENT

### Oxygen

When working in the home of someone on oxygen therapy, you must be aware of precautions while working around canisters of oxygen. Oxygen is delivered to patients in two ways: (1) tanks (cylinders) and (2) machine.

Oxygen tanks come in several sizes. Patients using a small amount of oxygen, for example, 1 or 2 liters per minute when needed, may have large green tanks of oxygen delivered to the home. Small oxygen tanks are used by patients for short trips outside the home. Patients using a larger amount of oxygen are usually supplied with a machine called an "oxygen concentrator." A concentrator pulls air from the environment and converts it into oxygen. Concentrators are more noisy than cylinders, but patients using them avoid:

- the need to store multiple tanks in the home
- the need to switch from an empty to a full tank

Use the following lists of home care aide dos and don'ts regarding oxygen use.

## *Do*

- Make certain that cylinders are stored in an upright position next to a wall.
- Follow up on patient education, if needed, such as the need to:
  1. place an oxygen sign in the entrance of the home
  2. not smoke around the oxygen or oxygen equipment
  3. be careful of the tripping hazard that oxygen tubing creates
- Observe the patient's breathing. If it seems to be more difficult than usual, ask the patient to discuss how he or she feels, and contact your supervisor or the nurse with your observations.
- Check the pressure spots when the patient wears a nasal cannula. These are behind the ears and at the

nostrils. Report any redness to the nurse. You may need to place small pieces of cotton between the ears and the tubing.

- Contact your supervisor with any questions you, the patient, or the family/caregiver have regarding the oxygen therapy.
- Remove all matches, ashtrays, and other smoking material from the room where oxygen is being administered.

## *Do Not*

- Do not lay cylinders on their sides or lean them in an unsteady manner.
- Do not use electrical equipment (e.g., electric razors, hair dryers) around the oxygen and tubing, because sparks can ignite the oxygen.
- Do not change the oxygen flow meter. Only the trained patient, caregiver, or professional staff members are permitted to make adjustments.
- Do not use any petroleum jelly product around the oxygen tubing.
- Do not use any talcum powder or perfumed objects around the patient with breathing problems.
- Do not drop or hit oxygen tanks.
- Do not use a gas stove if the patient, oxygen, or oxygen tubing is in or near the kitchen.

- Do not use woolen blankets; wool, silk, rayon, or nylon fabrics; or other materials that can cause static electricity.

## Hoyer Lift

Hoyer lifts are mechanical devices that assist caregivers in moving patients who might be unable to help themselves or who are very heavy for others to move safely. Hoyer lifts, when used according to instructions, are safe for the patient and prevent the home care aide from being hurt. When you assist the patient with transferring from bed to chair (or vice versa), follow this procedure:

1. Explain to the patient that you will use the lift to assist with the transfer.
2. Gather the Hoyer lift and any other items you may need (e.g., slippers, blanket).
3. Explain the procedure before you move the patient and also as you proceed with each step, if the patient's level of understanding or remembering is a problem.

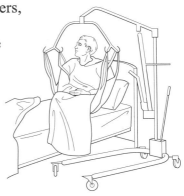

4. Place the chair close to the bed.
5. Elevate the bed and lower the side rail near you.
6. Assist the patient with turning away from you.
7. Place the Hoyer sling under the buttocks and back, gently tucking the excess sling under the patient.
8. Raise the side rail.
9. Assist the patient to roll over the excess sling toward you.
10. Move to the other side of the bed.
11. Gently pull the other half of the sling under to the other side of the patient.
12. Spread the feet of the lift to attain a wide base of support and place them under the bed.
13. Release the hydraulic valve and lower the trapeze portion of the lift to the patient. Take special care not to hit the patient with the trapeze portion.
14. Put the side rail closest to you down.
15. Place the metal hooks into the grooves of the trapeze.
16. Ask the patient to fold his or her arms across the chest for the lift.
17. Elevate the head of the bed.
18. While closely observing the security of the metal hooks within the grooves, pump the hydraulic handle to raise the patient above the bed.

19. Guide the patient over to the chair, taking care to clear the patient's path from the bed.
20. Position the patient over the seat of the chair.
21. Release the hydraulic lift and gently lower the patient onto the chair.
22. Remove the metal hooks and move the lift away from the patient.
23. Position the patient for comfort and security.

**Wheelchair**

In addition to routine wheelchairs, there are specialized wheelchairs built for patients with disabilities. Specialized wheelchairs have attachments made to help position the patient's upper body and/or failing extremities. Some are motorized and can travel at five to six miles per hour, which is rather fast inside a home. To assist a patient into a wheelchair:

1. Explain the procedure to the patient.
2. Gather equipment—wheelchair, gait belt, slippers, robe, etc.
3. Assist the patient to a sitting position.
4. Place the wheelchair at a 45° angle to the patient.
5. Lock the wheels.
6. Bend your knees and wrap your arms around the patient's back, just under the axilla. If desired, use a gait belt.

7. Count to three with the patient. At the count of "three," assist the patient to a standing position.
8. Pivot the patient to the wheelchair.
9. Ease patient down into the wheelchair, blocking the patient's knees from buckling with your knees.
10. Place the feet into the footrests.
11. Unlock the wheelchair, and roll patient to a location of choice.

## Bedside Commode

Some patients are able to sit up, stand, and pivot but for health reasons, or other reasons, are unable to walk to the bathroom. A portable toilet, called a bedside commode, can be rented and placed close to the patient. To assist the patient with the use of the bedside commode:

1. Explain the procedure to the patient.
2. Wash your hands.
3. Put on nonsterile gloves.
4. Gather equipment—bedside commode, toilet tissue, slippers, blanket, etc.
5. Assist the patient to a sitting position.
6. Place the bedside commode at a 45° angle to the patient.

7. Secure the commode from sliding with your foot.
8. Bend your knees and wrap your arms around the patient's back, just under the axilla. If desired, use a gait belt.
9. Put the patient's slippers on.
10. Count to three with the patient. At the count of "three," assist the patient to a standing position.
11. Pivot the patient to the bedside commode.
12. Ease patient down onto the bedside commode, blocking the patient's knees from buckling with your knees.
13. Cover the patient with the blanket.
14. Make sure the patient feels good (e.g., not lightheaded or dizzy).
15. If the patient is steady and has no dizziness, leave the room to provide privacy.
16. Assist the patient with wiping.
17. Return the patient to bed.
18. Empty commode and clean it.
19. Remove gloves.
20. Wash hands.

## Raised Toilet Seat

Patients with joint problems can benefit from an extension put over their commode to raise the seat. Raised toilet seats are most often used for tall patients and those with restricted movement of their hip joints, back, and/or knees. There are several types of raised toilet seats, each with different mechanisms to attach them to the commode. Each is packaged with directions. To place a raised toilet seat:

1. Gather equipment (raised toilet seat).
2. Wash hands.
3. Put on nonsterile gloves.
4. Raise the commode's actual seat and lid to the raised position.
5. Follow the manufacturer's guidelines. Common styles include
   - a solid plastic seat with a rim that fits into the bowl of the commode fixture
   - a partial plastic seat with solid plastic turns that screw the raised seat onto the lip of the commode bowl
   - a toilet seat with extended metal clamps
6. Test the security of the raised toilet seat placement by pushing against it with your hands. If it does not seem secure, tighten all connections or call your supervisor for instructions.
7. Remove gloves.
8. Wash hands.

## Urinal

Explain the procedure to the patient. The purpose is to provide a channel for waste elimination. Urinals are most often used by male patients; however, urinals are available for female patients also. Female urinals have a cupped opening rather than a round opening seen in male urinals.

1. Gather equipment—urinal, small towel for positioning.
2. Wash hands.
3. Put on nonsterile gloves.
4. Warm urinal with warm water and dry with a towel.
5. Provide for patient privacy.
6. Assist patient with placement of penis into urinal.
7. Secure urinal with small towel to avoid accidental spills.
8. Elevate head of bed as necessary.
9. Assist patient with urinal removal.
10. Assist patient with pericare, as necessary.
11. Empty urinal contents in commode.
12. Rinse urinal.
13. Remove gloves.
14. Wash hands.

## Bedpan

There are different kinds of bedpans made from either metal or hard plastic. Plastic bedpans are not cold, which is more comfortable for the patient. In addition to regular bedpans, there are also smaller bedpans, called fracture pans, used for patients with fractures and other musculoskeletal problems that make raising up painful, if not impossible. To help your patient with the bedpan placement:

1. Explain the procedure to the patient.
2. Wash your hands.
3. Put on nonsterile gloves.
4. Warm the metal bedpan with warm water and dry well.
5. Lower head of bed to flat position.
6. Assist patient onto bedpan, keeping narrow end of bedpan facing the foot of the bed in one of the following ways:
   a. Ask the patient to flex the knees with feet flat on the mattress.
   b. Help the patient to raise the hips by placing your hand under the small of his or her back, and position the bedpan under the buttocks. Or turn the patient on his or her side, place the bedpan in position, and roll the patient gently back onto the bedpan.

*or*

    a. Help the patient to turn away from you.
    b. Place the bedpan in the correct position encircling the buttocks and pubic area.
    c. Supporting the placement of the bedpan, instruct the patient to roll onto his or her back.

7. Elevate the head of the bed.
8. Place toilet tissue within the patient's reach, and provide patient with privacy.
9. Assist patient with bedpan removal.
10. Assist with perineal care.
11. Empty bedpan contents into commode and cleanse with antibacterial solution.
12. Replace equipment.
13. Remove gloves.
14. Wash hands.

## Tub Benches

Tub benches have plastic seats and a suction cup bottom on their four legs. They are placed inside the tub so the patient can sit for a bath or shower. Usually, patients using tub benches also have handheld shower extenders. Often they have grab bars on the outside wall of the tub or the wall of the tub enclosure. When using these types of aids, you need to encourage the patient to move carefully and make sure of sound footing before proceeding to the next step.

## Transfer Belts

Transfer belts are used to support the patient during transfers of positions. They help the helper by making the transfer process less difficult. To use a transfer belt during patient transfers:

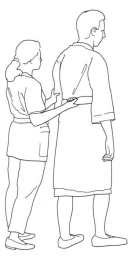

1. Instruct the patient about the procedure.
2. Place transfer belt around patient's waist:
   • Enter end of transfer belt into toothed side of buckle.
   • Fasten transfer belt securely and snugly around the waist so the belt does not slip up.
3. Position yourself in front of patient.
4. Wear gloves, if appropriate.
5. Place hands under patient's buttocks/upper thighs.
6. Slide patient to edge of chair or bed.
7. Fold patient's arms in front of the chest.
8. Help patient lean forward.
9. Reach around patient and grasp transfer belt at the back with your thumbs and fingers pointing up.

10. Assist patient to a standing position.
11. Have patient stand for 15 to 20 seconds while holding transfer belt.
12. Wait until patient feels balanced.
13. Pivot patient around to bed or chair.
14. Lower patient to bed or chair, using proper body mechanics.
15. Remove transfer belt from patient.

## Ambulation Aids

Patients can be assisted during ambulation by individuals or mechanical aids, such as canes, crutches, or walkers. When you are assisting a patient alone with ambulation:

1. Walk at the patient's side.
2. Place one arm behind the patient at waist level. Do not hold the waist if the patient is capable of walking. The purpose of this arm placement is to be prepared to support the patient in case he or she begins to fall.
3. Place your other hand on the patient's arm for support, if needed. (*Note:* If walking to the left of the patient, you will put your left hand on the patient's left upper arm and your right arm around the patient's back at waist level.)

When you and another person are assisting the patient:

1. One person should support the patient as described above.
2. The other person should support the patient's other arm by extending the lower arm, palm up, under the patient's lower arm, palm down.
3. Be aware of the length of the walk. If in doubt, place chairs at points along the way in case the patient needs to sit.

### *Canes*

Canes come in several forms. Most common canes have one point. These are called single-point canes. Quad canes provide more support for the patient. At the bottom of the cane is a plate with four legs. Hemi-canes have an armrest. Patients with hand problems place their arm inside the arm rest for support. Using this type of cane requires the strength of the arm rather than the strength of a hand. To assist the patient with ambulation using a cane, instruct the patient regarding the procedure, as follows:

- For walking on a flat surface:
  1. Hold cane close to body.
  2. Keep cane on uninvolved side.
  3. Keep length of step for each leg equal.
  4. Keep pace of each step equal.

- For stair climbing:
  1. Go up stairs with a railing by leading with the uninvolved (good) leg.
  2. Go up stairs without a railing by holding cane on uninvolved (good) side and leading with uninvolved (good) leg.
  3. Advance cane, then advance leg.
  4. Go down stairs with a railing by leading with the involved (bad) leg.
  5. Go down stairs without a railing by holding cane on uninvolved (good) side and leading with cane.
  6. Follow with involved (bad) leg, and then advance uninvolved (good) leg.
- In sitting down:
  1. Do not lean on cane. (This will help maintain balance and prevent patient falls.)
  2. Stand with back of legs against edge of chair seat.
  3. Grasp chair armrests with both hands.
  4. Lower body onto chair seat while supporting body weight with hands on armrests.

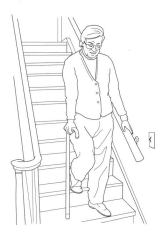

- In standing up:
  1. Do not lean on cane. (This will help maintain balance and prevent patient falls.)
  2. Grasp chair armrests with both hands.
  3. Scoot forward on the seat, placing involved (bad) foot and body slightly forward.
  4. Push hands against armrests to raise up from chair.

To help the patient stand:

1. Stand slightly behind patient and to the uninvolved side.
2. Place one foot between patient's feet and the other outside the uninvolved leg while instructing patient.

### *Crutches*

Crutches are used by individuals in need of support due to injured extremities. When accompanying patients as they walk with crutches, tell them to:

- Place crutches four to eight inches to the side of feet to form a three-point triangle.
- Relax shoulders.
- Stand straight.
- Instruct patient in ambulation on flat surfaces as follows:
  1. Move crutches forward six to eight inches.
  2. Lean forward.

3. Keep weight on hands.
4. Use three-point or four-point gait, as prescribed.
5. Maintain slow, even gait.
- Instruct patient in step climbing as follows:
  1. Use handrail with strongest arm.
  2. Place both crutches in hand away from railing.
  3. Push down on handrail.
  4. Step up with stronger leg.
  5. Raise weaker leg.
  6. Continue ascent, repeating above steps.
  7. Rest frequently.
- Instruct patient in step descending as follows:
  1. Hold handrail with stronger hand.
  2. Hold crutches in weaker hand.
  3. Advance weaker leg first, supported with crutches.
  4. Advance stronger leg to same step as weaker leg.
  5. Continue descent, repeating above steps.
  6. Rest frequently.

### *Walkers*

Walkers provide the patient with the most stability (other than the supportive assistance of two people). Patients using walkers can be assisted by reminders of the steps with using the walker:

1. Instruct patient about the procedure.
2. Put transfer belt around patient's waist per transfer of patient with transfer belt procedure, as appropriate.

3. Help patient to stand up, as follows:
   - Place walker to front of chair.
   - Have patient slide forward in chair.
   - Instruct patient to (1) place back of stronger leg against chair seat, (2) advance weaker leg, (3) place both hands on armrests, and (4) push up to a stand.
4. Help patient to grasp walker as follows:
   - Have patient support weight with stronger leg and opposite hand and grasp walker handgrip with free hand.
   - Have patient grasp other hand grip with other hand.
   - Assist patient to stand within walker and to hold handgrips firmly and evenly.
5. Help patient use walker, as follows:
   - Instruct individuals with one-sided weakness to (1) advance walker six to eight inches, (2) step forward with weaker leg, (3) support self on arms, and (4) follow weaker leg with stronger one.
   - Instruct individuals with equal strength in both legs to advance walker six to eight inches and step forward with either leg first.
   - Instruct individuals with use of only one leg to (1) advance walker six to eight inches, (2) swing onto weaker leg, and (3) support weight on hands.
6. Stand behind individual, toward the weaker leg.
7. Use transfer belt, if desired.

8. Instruct patient to take equal strides.
9. Instruct patient to sit down as follows:
   - Stand with back of stronger leg against front of chair.
   - Lift weaker leg slightly off floor.
   - Place walker directly in front.
   - Grasp chair armrests with the hand on same side as weaker leg.
   - Shift weight to stronger leg and hand grasping chair armrest.
   - Lower self into chair and slide backward.
10. Place walker beside the chair after patient is seated.
11. Remove transfer belt, if used.

## HOMEMAKING EQUIPMENT*

### Electric Equipment

#### *Stove/Oven*

Preparing hot meals or drinks for your patient is often done on the stove or in the oven. Most ovens are conventional. If you have never used the type of appliance in the patient's home, you should notify your supervisor. Cooking tips are located in Chapter 10.

---

*\*Source:* Reprinted with permission from ADVANTAGE Health Care Management Resources.

When using the stove top:

- Place pots and pans with the handles inward. Do not place them so that someone can hit the handle and knock the pot over, spilling hot contents.
- Use medium heat.
- Do not leave the room while cooking. If cooking something that must simmer, you may leave the room for short periods (two or three minutes) once you have brought the cooking temperature down to simmer.
- Use a pot or pan that is big enough for the food and utensils needed during the cooking process.
- Cook foods thoroughly.
- If the stove is gas powered, light the pilot carefully:
  1. Turn the knob to pilot if the stove is self-lighting. You will hear several clicks, and then the gas will ignite.
  2. Turn the knob until you hear a slight hiss of gas escaping in traditional gas stoves. Strike a match and place it close to the burner. The gas will ignite.

When using the oven:

- Use moderate temperatures recommended by a cookbook.
- Do not use the broiler unless you will stay at the oven during the broiling process.

- Use oven mitts to avoid burns.
- Open door, and then bend to transfer items in and out of the oven. This allows the initial blast of hot air to escape without burning you.
- Reduce the temperature by 25 degrees when using glass containers.
- When cooking at higher elevations, cook more slowly at lower temperatures.
- Cook foods thoroughly.

### Microwave Oven

Some of your patients may have microwave ovens. These ovens send intense heating waves into the food. Food cooks from the inside out and usually cooks much faster than with a traditional oven or stove top, depending on the size and wattage of the microwave. Microwaves are often used to reheat meals. If you are using the patient's microwave:

- Only use microwave-safe dishes.
- Do not place any foil or metal in the microwave.
- Ask the patient about the length of time the microwave takes to cook whatever you are preparing.
- Cover foods with plastic wrap or a paper towel to keep the warmth in.
- Stop during the cooking cycle to mix the food or turn the dish to allow even heating.

- Do not open the microwave door without first pushing the "pause" or "stop" button.
- At the end of the cycle, await the beeps that signal it is safe to open the door.
- Do not use the microwave for cooking if you, your patient, family, caregiver, or visitor have a pacemaker. No one with a pacemaker should come within 10 feet of the microwave when in use.

### Clothes Washer

When washing clothes:

1. Separate any contaminated/soiled laundry from other household clothing. Wash it in hot water and use bleach, if possible. (*Note:* Only use commercial bleach products that are approved for use with colors.)
2. Separate loads into like colors. Separate whites from colors.
3. Do not wash clothes that are new and have unstable colors with other garments.
4. Use hot water for undergarments, towels, and sheets.
5. Set the knob to the setting for the type of clothing (e.g., permapress, cottons).
6. Soak any badly soiled items for five minutes prior to washing. Use the soak cycle on the washer.

7. Put the detergent in the empty washer, and fill the tub to the required level with water.
8. Put bleach, if needed, into the bleach dispenser.
9. Allow the soap to dissolve in the water, and pull the knob out to stop the agitation.
10. Place the clothing in the tub.
11. Resume the wash cycle.
12. Do not open the lid until the machine stops.

### *Clothes Dryer*

Clothes dryers are routine appliances in today's home. Some of your elderly patients may have certain likes and dislikes about what is put in the clothes dryer rather than allowed to dry naturally. Check with the patient when you begin to work with him or her. When using a clothes dryer, keep the following in mind:

- Some materials cannot tolerate the extreme heat of a clothes dryer. Do not put sweaters or knits in the dryer.
- Towels and bed sheets can tolerate the hottest setting, while the delicate fabrics found in slacks, pants, blouses, and shirts do best with a cooler temperature.

Use the following procedure:

1. Place the clothing into the dryer after shaking it open from the tight spin cycle of the washer.

2. Turn the knob to the desired setting.
3. Place a fabric softener sheet in the dryer, if desired.
4. Close the door and push the knob in to start the dryer.
5. To avoid wrinkles, remove clothing as soon as it is dry.
6. Fold clothes and return them to their respective drawers or closet.

### *Dishwasher*

Dishwashers are an inexpensive alternative to washing dishes in the sink after every meal. Dishes, glasses, utensils, and pots or pans can be placed in the dishwasher after every meal and then washed when the washer is full. Some tips to help you with using a dishwasher follow:

1. Keep in mind that the water sprays up from the bottom of the dishwasher during the cycle.
2. Load the dishwasher keeping in mind the need to allow free flow of water from the bottom of the washer to the top, as follows:
   • Place cups, glasses, and small bowls in the upper rack with the open end facing downward.
   • Put utensils with the handle side up in the utensil holder. This prevents the need to touch the portion that is put into the mouth.

- Stack larger dishes in an alternating pattern on the bottom shelf.
- Place bowls, open end down, on the shelves.
- Do not wash plastic bowls in the dishwasher unless you know they are dishwasher safe. If in doubt, ask the patient.

3. Put detergent in the detergent canister.
4. Close and lock the door.
5. Turn the knob to the start position.
6. Push the knob in to start.
7. When the washer stops, it enters a drying cycle. Do not open during this cycle.
8. Once the dishwasher is through the drying cycle, it can be unloaded.
9. Look at each item as you remove it to make sure it is clean.
10. Return items to their shelves or cabinets.

### Vacuum Cleaner

Vacuum cleaners suck dust and other debris from the surface being cleaned. They come with a variety of attachments designed to get deep into the corners where dust can easily collect. The dust and debris is trapped in a bag inside the cleaner. When the vacuum cleaner is not picking up dust and debris as desired, it is a sign that the bag may need to be changed. Use the following procedure to vacuum:

1. Plug the electric cord into a grounded socket in the room you are vacuuming.
2. Using the brush attachments, clean the edges of the room first.
3. Detach the brush attachments, and move the furniture out of the way, if possible.
4. Using a back-and-forth motion, pass the cleaner over the carpet *slowly*.
5. Return furniture to its position, and continue in another section of the room.
6. Other attachments can be used to clean stuffed furniture, if desired.

## Nonelectric Equipment

### *Cleaning Furniture*

Routine furniture cleaning is done with a clean cloth and furniture spray. Furniture sprays moisten the cloth, which allows it to absorb more dust particles. To dust furniture in this manner:

1. Have several soft, clean cloths available. Replace a cloth when it becomes dirty.
2. Shake the furniture spray can well.
3. Spray the furniture spray directly onto the furniture from a distance of 8–12 inches.

4. Wipe the furniture until it is dry and shiny.
5. Make sure to get into all grooves and edges of each piece of furniture.

### *Cleaning Woodwork*

If desired, woodwork (moldings, windowsills, and doorways) can be cleaned with a mild household detergent, water, and clean cloths. Again, replace the cloths when dirty.

### *Cleaning Bathroom Fixtures*

Bathroom tubs and sinks can be cleaned with a commercial bathroom cleaner and wet cloth. Commodes should be cleaned with a disinfectant using a specially made toilet bowl brush.

### *Cleaning Kitchens*

There are special commercial products for cleaning the kitchen.

- Stove tops can be cleaned with a nonabrasive cleanser and wet cloth.
- Burner covers can be cleaned with an abrasive cleanser and steel wool pad.
- Ovens can be cleaned with an oven spray.
- Sinks can be cleaned with a nonabrasive cleanser.

- When cleaning countertops, remove all appliances, canisters, and knick-knacks. Clean the counter with mild soap and water.
- Clean appliances, canisters, and knick-knacks with a mild detergent preparation and wet cloth.
- Return all countertop items to their original location.

### *Floor Maintenance*

Floors should be swept or dry mopped and periodically washed with a commercial floor cleaner. Although scrubbing floors on hands and knees is the best method for floor care, homemakers are often not permitted to clean with such vigor. Using a commercial cleaner and wet mop works well for cleaning a patient's home.

# CHAPTER 9

# Reporting Requirements

## INTRODUCTION

As a home care aide, you must report information as it becomes known to you. Some information is gathered during interactions with the patient, family, and caregiver unit while other information pertains to you and your role as a home care aide. This chapter explains types of reporting and the information that you must convey to your supervisor.

## EMPLOYMENT-RELATED REPORTING

### Administrative Needs

The agency is required to keep current files that contain various forms, licenses, and documentation of events. You are responsible for giving your supervisor the information (written or oral) needed to keep your file up-to-date. Some of the necessary information varies from state to state. Generally, documents you must give to the agency include

- your certification card
- your certification test
- inservice education attended—both topics and hours
- copies of pretests and posttests
- documentation from the physician about physical results and vaccines you have received
- signed copies of annual performance evaluations
- signed copies of counseling forms
- in some agencies, copies of driver licenses and proof of vehicle insurance

You get some of these items throughout the year. It is your responsibility to remember to take a copy to your supervisor. Other items must be updated at intervals identified by the agency.

**Unplanned Absence from Work**

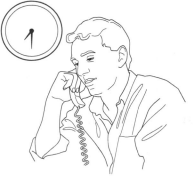

Both the patients and the agency count on you to arrive to work on time. Often you are the patients' only connection with the outside world, and they depend on you so they are able to stay at home. For that reason, unplanned absences from work should be kept to a minimum. Do *not* call in to take the day off if:

- Your family is sick. Find another person to help you with an ill child if necessary.
- You just are too tired to work or do not feel like working. You will leave people without needed care.
- The weather is bad. People have needs no matter what the weather is like. The expectation is that you will visit the patients as long as you can safely travel to and from their home.
- You want to extend a weekend, holiday, or vacation.

The only time you report off of work should be when:

- You are too ill to work.
- You have an infectious disease or illness.
- You have an injury that would prevent you from safely completing your patient care.
- There is an extreme emergency. (*Note:* Extreme emergencies include the approaching death of a close family member or being a victim of a recent crime.)

## How To Report Off of Work

When you report off of work, your supervisor or scheduler must do the following:

- Call other home care aides who are not working that day to find someone able to work in your place.
- Reschedule your patients' visits to another home care aide's schedule.
- Notify patients if a visit cannot be made.

To help with this process, it is very important for you to:

- Call your supervisor or scheduler as early as possible.
- Call the evening on-call nurse, if you know the night before that you will be unable to report to work the next day.
- Notify your supervisor or scheduler the day before if it seems clear that you will not be able to work the next day.

## Long-Term Illness and Disabilities

As discussed in Chapters 3 and 6, long-term illnesses and disabilities affect the patient's ability to function. These problems would also affect a home care aide's ability to function. Your employer must maintain confidentiality about any long-term illness or disability that you have. It would be helpful (although it is not required) for you to discuss any long-term illnesses and disabilities with your supervisor. In case you need to call in absent from work, your supervisor will have a better understanding and be more supportive of your health-related needs.

The Americans with Disabilities Act was passed to make sure that employers do everything that is reasonable and possible to keep Americans with disabilities functioning in the work world. If you have a disability, your employer should work with you in scheduling patients to whom you are able to provide care, for example:

- If you are highly allergic to cats and dogs your supervisor or the scheduler can arrange for you to visit only homes without these domestic animals.
- If you have a muscular problem with your back, your supervisor or scheduler can schedule you to visit patients who are not in need of lifting.

On the other hand, if every one of the agency's home care aides has back problems, it may not be able to accommodate these needs in scheduling because there will always be patients in need of lifts and assistance.

## Late for Work

If you awake to an emergency (e.g., a big snowfall, an ill child, a dead battery in the car) and will need to take action before going to work, you must notify your supervisor or the scheduler as early as possible. They will need to know

- that you will be late
- an approximate time that you will be able to report to your first patient
- the nature of the problem
- whether or not you have contacted any of your patients

Due to the busy time in the mornings in home care agencies, supervisors and schedulers appreciate your taking the time to call your first patient to tell him or her that you are going to be late and that the office will call later with any changes.

## Asking for Time Off

One of the benefits of working is the ability to take some time off from the job. Full- and part-time employees usually receive paid holiday and vacation days. Temporary pool or prn (if needed) staff usually are not obligated to work specific days and can select their own schedule. If possible, when requesting time off:

- Give at least two weeks' notice.
- Remember that time off is scheduled either on a first-come, first-approved basis or by seniority.

- Do not buy expensive tickets and schedule a room on the cruise until you have cleared the time off with your employer.
- Follow the procedure set up within your agency.

## AGENCY-RELATED REPORTING

In Chapter 6 you were told diagnosis-specific items to be reported to your supervisor. Agencies often require their home care aides to always report the following.

### Changes in Patient Status

- ability to ambulate, transfer, and care for self
- change in mental alertness (e.g., forgetfulness, confusion)
- comments about not taking medicine or not following the physician's orders
- complaints
- decline in ability to care for self
- environmental hazards or concerns
- falls
- family/caregiver events (e.g., death, caregiver moves)
- fever
- increased or new development of pain

- lack of necessary supplies
- progress of patient in ability to care for self
- rashes
- red areas or bed sores
- refusal of care
- reports leading you to believe that the patient is able to get out of the house
- requests for care that is not on the care plan that the nurse designed
- shortness of breath
- suspected or observed abuse or neglect
- changes in vital signs:
  1. blood pressure greater than 150/90
  2. pulse less than 60 or greater than 90
  3. respirations fewer than 12 or greater than 24
  4. temperature below 97°F or greater than 101°F

## Incident Reports

Some of the items above are reported both orally and in writing. An incident report is used for reporting:

- any event that leads to personal injury (patient, caregiver, agency visitors, agency staff)
- any event leading to property damage
- any potential hazard

Incident reports are reviewed by someone in the agency, and they provide valuable information about opportunities for improvement or processes that may need to be changed to give a higher quality of care. When completing an incident report:

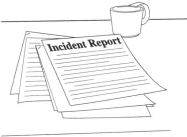

- Complete the report as soon as possible when the event is the most clear in your memory.
- Be thorough in what you write.
- Describe the event in detail. (You may need this to refresh your memory if called into court.)
- Be clear in what you write.
- Have your supervisor read the report and make comments.
- Follow through with appropriate suggestions your supervisor makes.
- Write legibly. *You* may have to read this some day!
- Submit your report within 24 hours of the incident.

**Adherence to Care Plan**

The care plan serves as a report of the nurse's assessment about the patient. It lists the actions that the nurse believes you must perform for the patient. Following the care plan is very important. As a home care aide, you are not permitted to develop a plan for the patient. The nurse is mandated by law to do this for you. Your documentation links you to following the care plan. It may be looked at for several reasons:

- *Legal purposes.* It shows a lawyer what you did for that patient during that particular visit. It also is a legal document stating that you did what you were supposed to do.
- *Reimbursement purposes.* It shows the payer what you did for the patient so that the payer can evaluate whether the service provided is a reimbursable service.
- *Regulation purposes.* It shows the surveyor from the department of health what you did. The surveyor compares what you wrote down that you did to what the nurse asked you to do. If there are any differences, the surveyor wants to know why.
- *Quality purposes.* It shows the surveyor from the accrediting body the way the agency plans for the patient and how staff talk with each other and follows through with their care.

## Documentation of Care

Writing down your activities makes a written report of what was done during a patient visit. Use the following tips as you document:

- Take credit for all that you do in the home by documenting it.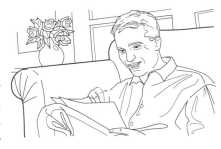
- Compare your documentation to what you were directed to do by the nurse.
- Document about *every* item on the care plan.
- Document at the visit or immediately upon leaving the home.
- Remember the limits of your certification. Do not take over documentation of another discipline's area.
- Write legibly.
- Document in blue or black ink. Never use pencil.
- Make corrections by striking a single line through the incorrect entry and placing your initials and the date above.
- *Never* use liquid correction fluid (Wite-Out).
- Write in sentences.
- If you forgot to write something, do not cram it in. Write it at the end as an "Addendum to the documentation."
- *Never* tamper with a clinical record. Tampering is
    1. adding to a clinical note at a later date without indicating that it is a late entry

2. placing inaccurate information in a record
3. purposefully omitting information
4. rewriting or altering the documentation
5. destroying clinical record notes or other documents
6. adding to someone else's notes without indicating your identity and the date
- Include the following in documentation:
  1. information about the patient's current condition
  2. any information that you reported (What did you report to whom?)
  3. reasons why this patient requires ongoing care and support
  4. changes in the care plan that you received an oral approval for over the phone
  5. patient/caregiver response to care

## Timely Submission of Documentation

Other documents serve as reports for surveyors and any other reviewer of the agency. Unless your supervisor tells you differently, you should submit items within the time frames outlined in Table 9–1.

## Environmental Concerns

Environmental concerns need to be reported to your agency. Some examples include fire hazards, faulty elec-

**Table 9–1** Suggested Timelines for Documentation Submission

| Item | Submission Deadline |
| --- | --- |
| 1. Daily patient documentation | As soon as possible, at least weekly |
| 2. Copy of certification card | Upon receipt |
| 3. Copy of driver's license | Upon receipt |
| 4. Copy of vehicle insurance | Upon receipt |
| 5. Proof of TB testing | Annually or semiannually, depending on organization's location/patient mix |
| 6. Copy of physical | Per organizational policy |

trical wiring, and unsafe use of oxygen. If you are in a patient's home and observe any environmental problems, call your supervisor or the patient's nurse to report your concerns. Do not forget to document your actions in your patient daily note.

Environmental concerns pertaining to the agency should be reported to your supervisor. Examples include outdated or partially filled fire extinguishers, icy patches in the parking lot, and improper storage of hazardous waste. In some cases an incident report of these findings is written.

## Customer Complaints

Customers who complain to you are complaining to the agency. It is good when customers voice their complaints, because those who complain

- are giving the agency a chance to "make it better"
- would rather continue receiving care from your agency
- are being honest with you

The alternative is for the patient with a complaint to call your agency and cancel services. In this case, human nature often takes over and the patient is likely to complain about your agency to others in the community. This is very harmful to the agency.

When patients complain:

- Ask questions to better understand their concerns.
- Tell your supervisor about the complaint.
- Write a written report on a complaint form or incident form, as directed by your supervisor.

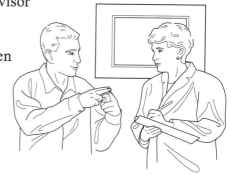

## Some Signs of Abuse and Neglect

Chapter 5 (Exhibit 5–1) lists the signs of patient abuse and neglect. Whenever you suspect that a patient is being either abused or neglected, you must report your concerns to your supervisor. The agency is required by law to report any concerns to the appropriate agency:

- If the patient is a child, concerns are reported to the Children and Youth Agency.
- If the patient is an adult, concerns are reported to Adult Protective Services.

Sometimes health care workers just are not sure and do not want to falsely accuse someone if it is not true. If you find yourself unsure about a situation, it may be helpful to understand the following:

- Just because a situation of possible abuse/neglect is reported does not mean that the individual is guilty.
- The workers from these protective services are well trained in how to approach the patient and caregivers without making them feel guilty.
- For the patient, it would be better if you over-report than do not report abusive or neglectful behavior.
- Your supervisor will support you and take some of the burden of reporting from you.

## Interdisciplinary Care Team

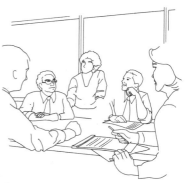

As part of the team you will have valuable input for all of the other disciplines at one point or another. It is important that you follow the communication lines established by the agency. Patient information that should be reported to other members of the interdisciplinary care team includes the following:

- *Physical therapist:* Changes in ability to ambulate, transfer, pivot, stand, and endure these activities; changes in weight-bearing status. In my agency, the person I need to contact is _____ .
- *Occupational therapist:* Changes in ability to perform activities of daily living; changes in weight-bearing status or activity. In my agency, the person I need to contact is _____ .
- *Speech-language pathologist:* Changes in ability to speak, write, or read; changes in swallowing, such as choking or improved swallowing. In my agency, the person I need to contact is _____ .

- *Nurse:* Changes in patient status. In my agency, the person I need to contact is _____ .
- *Physician:* Any changes necessitating a change in orders. In my agency, the person responsible for getting physician orders is _____ .
- *Social worker/counselor:* Any changes in support system, coping, level of mental alertness, or financial status. In my agency, the person I need to contact with these issues is _____ .
- *Bereavement coordinator:* Impending death or family/caregiver issues. In my agency, the person I need to contact with these issues is _____ .
- *Medical director:* Any issue necessitating intervention with other physicians, physician orders, or agency medical policies. In my agency, the person I need to contact with these issues is _____ .
- *Dietitian:* Any nutritional issue having to do with the type of intake or losing or gaining excessive weight. In my agency, the person I need to contact with these issues is _____ .

Your role in communication is important. Follow the principles for communication outlined in Chapter 4 to enhance your reporting skills.

# CHAPTER 10

# Resources and Useful Information

This chapter contains important information for you to reference from personal and work-related perspectives. It is subdivided into

- Important Information about the Patient
- Community Resources
- Important Information about Your Role as a Home Care Aide
- Procedures for Care Delivery

## IMPORTANT INFORMATION ABOUT THE PATIENT

### Nutritional Needs*

#### *I&O (Intake & Output)*

At times, the home care aide must measure the patient's intake and output. Patient conditions that warrant this measuring include

---

*Source:* Reprinted with permission from *The Home Health Aide Educator,* ADVANTAGE Health Care Management Resources Press.

- fluid retention
- kidney disease
- urinary tract disorders
- heart disease
- nutritional problems

For intake and output measurement, liquids are defined as anything that is liquid at room temperature, including beverages, ice cream, gelatin, popsicles, and soups. The liquids taken in by the patient must be tracked and measured in like amounts, for example, cc's, ounces, or cups. Use the box of equivalencies to help you measure in the selected "like amounts."

| Cups | Ounces | cc's |
|------|--------|------|
| 1/4  | 2      | 60   |
| 1/2  | 4      | 120  |
| 3/4  | 6      | 180  |
| 1    | 8      | 240  |
| 2    | 16     | 480  |

Liquid output is also tracked and measured. Liquid output includes

- urine
- diarrhea
- vomitus
- wound drainage

Measuring devices used for intake include measuring cups and content ounces. Measuring devices used for output include basins and pans to catch the output and dedicated measuring devices, such as calibrated cups or containers.

### Special Diets

*Diabetic Diet.* This is a balanced diet with daily servings from the six food groups: breads, meats, milks, vegetables, fruits, and fats. The patient's physician instructs the patient on the number of calories and number of servings from each food group that are required for the patient's sex, weight, and activity level. A copy of the diet should be in the patient's home. If not, contact your supervisor.

Diabetic patients should follow these guidelines:

- Eat at the same times every day.
- Do not eat anything with concentrated sugar (e.g., cake, pie, candy).
- Eat a variety of foods within each food group.
- Bake, broil, or boil instead of fry food.

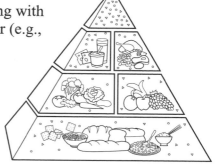

*NAS Diet.* A no added salt (NAS) diet is just that, a diet where no salt is added at the table. In addition, the cook should not add more salt during cooking to make up for not being able to add salt at the table. Patients on a no added salt diet also should avoid salty foods such as

- pickles
- olives
- mustard
- processed cheese
- lunch meats
- bacon
- ham
- sauerkraut
- chips
- pretzels
- canned soups and vegetables

*Low-Sodium Diet.* A low-sodium diet is used by people with kidney and severe heart problems. Patients on a low-sodium diet cannot add salt at the table, plus they must count the milligrams of sodium in the food they eat throughout the day. The physician will tell the patient how many milligrams of sodium he or she can have in a day, usually 2000 (also called a 2 gram sodium diet) or 1000 (also called a 1 gram sodium diet). It is important for the cook to read the content labels and add up all the milligrams of sodium.

*Cardiac/Low-Fat Diet.* Low-fat, cardiac healthy diets limit the amount of fat grams consumed by the patient. Patients must limit their intake of certain foods:

- red meat: three servings (3–4 ounces/serving) per week
- eggs: two per week
- high-fat foods (e.g., foods with butter, oil, lard, shortening)

Use the following tips to limit fat:

- Prepare red meat no more than twice a week.
- Trim fat from meat before cooking.
- Remove skin from chicken, turkey, and other fowl before cooking.
- Pan fry using a nonstick pan and cooking spray.
- Bake, broil, or poach food. Microwaving is also good.
- Baste meats with nonfat liquids such as lemon juice, defatted beef or chicken broth, or wine.
- Let sauces and soups cool, and skim the layer of fat off the top.
- Substitute skim milk for regular milk and cream.

In addition to the above, read the labels of foods to see how much fat they have. Fat is measured in grams, and a low-fat diet has less than 20 grams of fat per day. Also, if you have a choice between unsaturated or saturated fats, use the unsaturated fat. Saturated fat is solid at room temperature, like lard, shortening, or butter. It can clog up the arteries and veins quickly. The other kind of fat, unsaturated fat, is broken down more easily so the body can get rid of it.

*High-Fiber Diet.* High-fiber diets help patients have regular and soft bowel movements. Foods with high fiber include

- whole-grain cereals and breads
- fruits, such as prunes, apples, apricots, peaches, dates, and figs
- green, leafy vegetables

*High-Calorie Diet.*\* Patients put on high-calorie diets need to gain weight. The physician will order the number of calories the patient should have on a daily basis. A balanced diet can be supplemented with

- high-calorie commercial beverages
- homemade milkshakes between meals
- high concentrated sugar products (e.g., pie, cake, soda, candy)

---

\**Source:* Reprinted with permission from *The Home Health Aide Educator,* ADVANTAGE Health Care Management Resources Press.

To help these patients take in more calories, the home care aide should encourage them to eat two more bites with every meal or drink one more ounce of high-calorie beverages. The patient should not be forced to eat or drink to the point of vomiting.

*High-Protein Diet.** High-protein diets are used for patients during the healing process (e.g., for patients with burns or open wounds, postoperative patients). Foods with high protein include

- meats
- fish
- poultry
- milk and dairy products (not butter)
- soybeans and other legumes

*Low–Vitamin K Diet.* This diet is used by patients taking oral blood thinners. The patient should not eat large quantities of foods with vitamin K, because it alters the blood-thinning effect of oral blood thinners. Vitamin K is found in the following foods:

---

*Source: Reprinted with permission from *The Home Health Aide Educator,* ADVANTAGE Health Care Management Resources Press.

- dark green, leafy vegetables
- wheat, rye, alfalfa
- cabbage
- spinach
- cauliflower
- green tomatoes
- peas
- rose hips
- yogurt
- kelp

If the patient eats varying amounts of these foods from day to day, the physician may have difficulty finding the right dose of the blood thinner. This puts the patient at risk for severe bleeding or clotting.

*Bland Diet.* Bland diets are used for patients with stomach problems or patients who have not been eating and are now starting to eat. Patients on a bland diet

- should not eat spicy, hot foods
- should not eat foods that are digested slowly (e.g., red meats)
- should not eat high fat concentrated condiments and foods (e.g., gravy, cream sauces)
- can eat non–cream-based soups
- can have potatoes, breads, and grain products, such as pastas

*Liquid Diet.* Liquid diets are used after a bout of not eating due to influenza or inability to digest. Liquids are considered anything that at room temperature would be liquid in consistency, including

- beverages
- gelatins
- popsicles
- soup broth
- ice cream, frozen yogurt
- puddings

*Pureed Diet.* Pureed diets allow the patient with swallowing problems to get the taste and nutrition of regular foods in a thickness they are able to swallow. To puree foods:

- Use a food processor or blender.
- Add some broth or milk to blenderize it to a thick liquid consistency.
- Serve food at the appropriate temperature.

In addition to pureed foods, the patient is able to take in thick liquids such as puddings and ice cream.

### Meal Planning

Planning for patients' meals means learning about

- their special diet, if any
- their food likes and dislikes
- their preferences

Planning is best done prior to food shopping for the week. Only items that will be needed during the week should be purchased.

### *Food Shopping*

When shopping for food, the home care aide should do the following:

- Discuss the grocery needs with the patient.
- Take the money from the patient. (Do not get the money yourself. If necessary, hand the wallet to the patient.)
- Prepare a list of items needed.
- Purchase only what is on the list.
- Read labels for ingredients that the patient cannot have due to a special diet.
- Compare the cost with the amount, and purchase the best buy. Buy meats, dairy products, and fresh fruits and vegetables close to home.
- Be careful not to let meat juices drip onto other groceries in the cart.
- Use a cooler to carry cold groceries home if it will take more than 30 minutes.

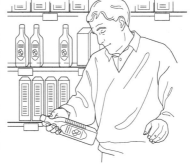

- Immediately give the patient the sales slips and change upon returning.

### Food Storage

- Store cold foods at 40°F.
- Store frozen foods at 0°F.
- Never refreeze.
- Put cooked food in the refrigerator or freezer immediately.

### Food Preparation

- Never thaw meat at room temperature or in warm water.
- Thaw meat in the refrigerator or in the microwave.
- Wash all utensils and cutting boards with soap and water after using them.
- Clean counters thoroughly after meal preparation.
- Cook meat well, that is, until juice runs clear and temperature reaches 165°F for 15 seconds.

### Serving Food

- Keep hot foods hot.
- Keep cold foods cold.
- Do not eat foods that have been left out of refrigeration for more than two hours.

**Skin Care**

When caring for skin, the home care aide must do the following:

- Observe the skin condition.
- Plan the followthrough.
- Provide the needed care.

If a patient's skin is dry and no open areas are observed:

- Use soap only for pericare and underarms.
- Use a commercial bath lotion in the bath water.
- Apply lotion to the skin after the bath.

If red areas are observed but no open areas:

- After bathing, gently massage the area with moisturizing lotion.
- Educate the patient and caregiver about the importance of frequent position changes.
- Communicate the information to the nurse/supervisor.

If open areas are observed:

- Cleanse the area gently with a soft cloth and water.
- Discard water and use a different cloth to continue with the bath.

- Do not apply anything to the area.
- Communicate the information immediately to the nurse/supervisor.

## First Aid

You may need to give first aid when you least expect it. You should know what steps to take in the event of a problem requiring first aid.

### Insect Stings

1. Observe the patient for signs of difficulty with breathing or absence of a heart rate.
2. Remove the stinger.
3. Call your supervisor to report the sting and follow his or her directions.
4. If the patient has signs of breathing difficulties, call for an ambulance to take the patient to the physician's office or the emergency department of the local hospital.

### Bleeding—Severe

1. Stop the bleeding by applying pressure directly over the bleeding area with a clean cloth.
2. If an arm or leg is bleeding, raise the extremity to decrease the flow of blood.
3. Ask someone to call for help (e.g., ambulance).

4. Stay with the person until help arrives and your services are no longer needed.

## Cuts and Abrasions

1. Clean the wound with mild antibacterial soap and water.
2. Apply Band-Aid.
3. Notify your supervisor and/or the patient's nurse.

## Choking

If the patient cannot talk, breathe, or cough and *is alert:*

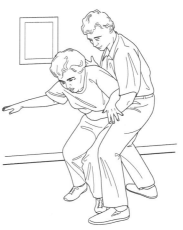

1. Stand behind the patient.
2. Place your arms around the patient's waist.
3. Give four upward thrusts on the stomach.
4. Bend patient over.
5. Give four upward thrusts between the shoulder blades.
6. Assess for breathing. If no breathing, repeat the above steps until the airway is open.

If the patient is *not* alert:

1. Lay patient down.
2. Turn patient's head to the side.
3. Place your index finger into the mouth and scoop out any contents.
4. Attempt to breath into the patient.
5. If you cannot get air to go in:
   - Straddle the patient by sitting over him or her.
   - Place your palms on the patient's abdomen.
   - Give four upward thrusts.
   - Position yourself to the side of the patient.
   - Roll the patient toward you.
   - Lean over the patient and give four upward thrusts between the shoulder blades.
6. Repeat these steps until the airway is open.

In either situation, ask someone to call for help, and stay with the patient until help arrives or your services are no longer needed.

### *Not Breathing*

1. Check to determine whether the patient is breathing by placing your cheek about one inch above the mouth and nose.
2. If the patient is not breathing:
   - Use your protective CPR mask.
   - Begin artificial breathing.

### *Not Breathing, No Heart Rate*

1. Initiate CPR, if trained.
2. Ask someone to call for help (ambulance).
3. Continue CPR and stay with the patient until help arrives and your services are no longer needed.

### *Burns—Minor*

1. Place burned area in cold water.
2. Report situation to supervisor and/or patient's nurse.

### *Burns—Major*

1. Do not remove patient's clothing, since it may remove the protective skin.
2. Put the burned part of the body in cold water as soon as possible. Do not use ice.
3. If burns are deep, cover the burns as soon as possible with a sterile or clean white cloth or gauze.
4. Call for help.
5. Stay with the patient until help arrives and your services are no longer needed.
6. Keep the patient alert by talking with him or her.

### *Swallowing Poison*

1. Give the patient a glass of milk.
2. Call the poison control center in your area (phone _____), or call the local hospital's emergency department (phone _____) for help.

3. If the patient should vomit, save and send it to the emergency department with the patient.

### *Inhalation of Poisons or Smoke*

1. Move the patient to a well-aired place (outside if possible).
2. Call the poison control center in your area (phone _____), or call the local hospital's emergency department (phone _____) for help.
3. Observe the patient for difficulty breathing.
4. Stay with the patient until help arrives and your services are no longer needed.
5. Follow the procedure outlined in Chapter 7 to report a fire.

## Skin Ulcer Assessments

As you observe patients' skin, be aware that there are different kinds of ulcerations or bedsores, as follows:

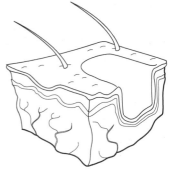

Dissected View of Stage III Ulcer

• Stage I—Redness that does not dissipate after 30 minutes of pressure relief.

- Stage II—Partial thickness loss of skin (may be a blister). Wound base is pink and painful.
- Stage III—Full thickness tissue loss that may result in some necrosis, sinus tract formation, exudate, and possibly infection. Wound is usually not painful.
- Stage IV—Deep tissue involvement into the fascia, possibly the muscle, joint, and bone. Wound is usually not painful.

As a home care aide, your responsibilities are to:

- Gently massage the area around Stage I ulcers.
- Report ulcers of any other stage immediately to your supervisor.

## Assessment of Edema (Fluid Retention)

If you want to know if your patient is retaining fluid, you can push the skin in gently, then release and observe what happens. Edema is measured in pluses (+), as follows:

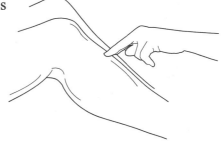

+1—Skin blanches to touch and immediately returns to normal color when pressure is released.

+2—Skin blanches to touch, and an indentation is barely palpable.

+3—Skin indents to touch and remains indented for up to 10 seconds.

+4—Skin indents to touch and remains indented for more than 10 seconds.

As a home care aide, you would report any signs of edema to your supervisor or the patient's nurse.

## COMMUNITY RESOURCES

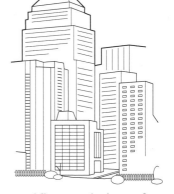

Good sources for information about community resources in your area are

- the phone book
- the United Way
- the Area Agency on Aging
- associations targeted to specific populations, for example, The AIDS Project, The Lung Association

Some common community resources for patients, families, and caregivers are listed in Exhibit 10–1.

**Exhibit 10–1** Community Resources for Patients, Families, and Caregivers

| | |
|---|---|
| The United Way | This organization collects money and distributes it to community agencies that operate to help people without collecting a profit. As such, it is a good place to learn about some of the resources available. |
| The Area Agency on Aging | This agency oversees services for those over age 59 in the community. It has various programs in different areas, such as homemaker care, transportation services, and grocery shopping. Each is mandated to cover adult protective services. |
| Family and Children's Services | This agency oversees social services for parental-child issues such as abuse and neglect. It also offers parenting classes and other educational resources. |

*continues*

**Exhibit 10–1** continued

| | |
|---|---|
| The AIDS Project | This resource oversees and advocates for services for patients diagnosed with acquired immune deficiency syndrome. |
| The American Cancer Society<br>The American Council for the Blind<br>The American Diabetes Association<br>The American Heart Association<br>The American Lung Association<br>The American Parkinson's Disease Association<br>The National Association of the Deaf<br>The National Institute on Alcohol Abuse and Alcoholism<br>The National Institute on Allergy and Infectious Disease<br>The National Institute on Arthritis and Musculoskeletal Diseases<br>The National Institute on Deafness and Other Communication Disorders<br>The National Institute on Digestive and Kidney Diseases<br>The National Kidney Foundation<br>The National Institute on Drug Abuse<br>The National Multiple Sclerosis Society<br>The National Osteoporosis Foundation<br>The National Stroke Association | There are community resources in many areas with information and support for specific targeted illnesses. If there is no local chapter in your area, you can contact the United Way for information about the national organization for that illness. National organizations provide educational materials and information about the closest agency to your locale. National organizations can also assist with information to form a local chapter in your area. |

At times you may need to talk with someone about personal situations. Keep the community resources in Exhibit 10–1 in mind, for they can be helpful to you, as well as to a family member or caregiver. Other resources useful to home care aides appear in Exhibit 10–2.

## IMPORTANT INFORMATION ABOUT YOUR ROLE AS A HOME CARE AIDE

### The Home Care Aide's Role during a Survey*

Home care and hospice agencies have surveys at various points in time. The Department of Health surveys the agency for compliance with government regulations, while accreditors such as the Joint Commission on Accreditation of Healthcare Organizations or CHAP (National League of Nursing, Community Health Assessment Program), survey organizations for compliance with quality-related standards. In some states, the accreditors have permission to survey agencies instead of the Department of Health. These surveyors may visit the agency every one to three years.

---

*\*Source:* Reprinted with permission from *The Home Health Aide Educator,* ADVANTAGE Health Care Management Resources Press.

**Exhibit 10–2** Community Resources for the Home Care Aide

| *To find out more about . . .* | *Call* |
|---|---|
| Infections/communicable disease in your county | County health department |
| Information about FDA-approved products | FDA's Consumer Hotline at 1-301-443-1240 |
| Food preparation | USDA's Meat and Poultry Hotline at 1-800-535-4555 |
| The Americans With Disabilities Act | House Document Room Room B 18 Annex 2 Washington, DC (1-202-225-3456) |
| Personal guidance and counseling services | County mental health department |

To help the agency succeed in the survey:

- Make sure all of your documentation and reports are turned in on time. If you are late returning an evaluation, the surveyor may say that your supervisor never did the evaluation because it is not in your personnel file.
- Dress in uniform.
- Wear your name badge.
- Act professionally in the presence of the surveyor.

The surveyor will want to observe the care given by different staff. You may be selected as one of these staff members. The surveyor will want to talk with you or observe you while you care for a patient. Here are a few tips to help you if you are selected to talk with the surveyor:

- Remain calm.
- Feel good inside because you give good care.
- If you are unsure of the answer to the question, either ask the surveyor to restate the question so you can understand it or state that you are unsure and would check with your supervisor.
- Represent your agency positively. Do not "bad mouth" anyone to the surveyor.
- Answer the questions asked by the surveyor, but do not talk on and on about other issues unless asked.

If you are selected to make a patient visit with the surveyor:

- Remain calm.
- Block out the fact that you are being observed.
- Remember to use universal precautions.
- Talk with your patient just as you would normally.
- If you notice any hazards in the home, discuss your concerns with the patient. Do not ignore an identified problem.

## Ethical Dilemmas

Ethical dilemmas are situations that come up through the course of working in home care or hospice that make you feel unsure about how to proceed. Some examples of ethical dilemmas are the following:

- The patient insists that you take a family heirloom because you have a special relationship.
- The patient refuses to take her medicine even though it means that her heart will beat funny and she will die. The patient's son insists that you force the patient to take her medicine.
- The patient refuses to get help or move to a nursing home. He no longer meets your agency's policy for continuation of service, but if you discharge him, he will be in worse shape.

To solve ethical issues, most agencies

- have committees that discuss the situation and come to a solution
- want input from the field staff, including the home care aide
- include the perspective of the patient and family/ caregiver, if applicable

If you become aware of any ethical dilemmas, you must report them to your supervisor.

## Map Reading

A job in home health care means that you need to travel in unfamiliar places. Directions to patients' homes are usually provided. If the directions are not complete enough to route you from home to home, you might want to obtain a map. Most counties have inexpensive street maps for all areas. Once you have a map in front of you, you need to:

- Determine where you are.
- Determine which direction you are facing.
- Find your location on the map.
- Find your destination on the map.

After noting these important locations on the map, you can identify the streets and roads you need to take. It is a good idea to list the streets in sequence of use from your location to the

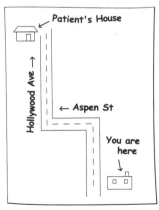

patient's home. If the map is held so that the streets in front of you are up in the map, you can also add to your list which direction you need to turn at each street. Until you become good at reading a map, you may want to try to keep the map aligned in the direction of your route so that the map and the direction you should turn correspond. Then you would need to:

- Turn left when the street you need is to the left of you.
- Turn right when the street you need is to the right of you.

All maps have legends that give the number of miles per inch. If the ratio is two miles per inch, you can write down approximately how long you need to travel on each road. Legends also give you the key to map reading. For example, bold lines might represent divided highways, regular lines might represent city streets, and red lines might represent interstates.

## What To Do If You Are in an Auto Accident

If you are involved in an accident while traveling:

1. Remain calm.
2. Stop and think: Do you smell gas?
   - If no, there is not a need to get out of the vehicle if you are unable.

- If yes: (1) Turn the key in the ignition off. (2) Remove the key from the ignition. *Note:* Do not attempt to restart car. (3) Get out of the vehicle as soon as possible to avoid being in the vehicle during a possible explosion or fire.

3. Determine whether you are able to get out of the vehicle:
   - Can you move?
   - Do you have severe pain anywhere?
   - Does the door open?

4. Pull the vehicle off the road unless:
   - You are unable.
   - The vehicle will not move.
   - Moving the vehicle will destroy important evidence showing who was at fault.

5. If you are able, get out of the vehicle.

6. Ask someone to notify the police.

7. Find out if the other driver or any passengers are injured.

8. Share information with the other driver:
   - name
   - address
   - insurance company name
   - insurance agent name
   - insurance policy number

9. Explain what happened to the police officer. Do not admit to or discuss any wrongdoing.

10. Once the police are finished, call your supervisor.
11. Call your insurance agent as soon as possible.
12. Take a few minutes to collect yourself before continuing with your day.

## Medications

In most states, home care aides are not permitted, by law, to give any medication to patients. It is important to understand what is included under the heading of "medications." Medications include

- pills prescribed by a physician
- over-the-counter pills, including vitamins
- injectable medications, such as insulin
- ointments, salves, and medicated lotions
- inhaled medications, such as oxygen and inhalers
- medicated eye, ear, and nose drops

As a home care aide, you should never administer medications unless your supervisor approves doing so. If necessary, you may remind the patient of the time and place medications within the patient's reach.

## PROCEDURES FOR CARE DELIVERY*

In addition to the procedures in previous chapters, the following procedures are pertinent to the home care aide.

---

*Source: Procedures used with permission from ADVANTAGE Health Care Management Resources.

**Diapering**

*Infant*

1. Change infant diapers whenever they are wet to the point that urine is wetting the skin surface.
2. Wash your hands.
3. Put on nonsterile gloves.
4. Gather supplies: clean diaper, diapering wipes or damp cloth, baby powder.
5. Lay the infant on a safe surface.
6. Talk with the infant throughout the procedure and play age-appropriate games, such as peek-a-boo.
7. Remove the soiled diaper.
8. Discard diaper into diaper pail.
9. Thoroughly clean the infant's lower abdomen, genitalia, and buttocks.
10. Observe for signs of diaper rash or excoriation. If present, call your supervisor when possible.
11. Dry the area and apply baby powder.
12. Place clean diaper under buttocks.
13. Pull the front of the diaper through the legs and up to cover the lower abdomen.
14. Secure the diaper using tape (disposable diapers) or safety pins, pointing downward (cloth diapers).
15. Replace clothing.
16. Return infant to a safe location.
17. Discard disposable wipes or wash washcloths and soiled cloth diaper.

18. Remove gloves.
19. Wash hands.
20. Document procedure.

### *Adult*

1. Change adult diapers after the patient urinates or has a bowel movement.
2. Wash your hands.
3. Put on nonsterile gloves.
4. Gather supplies: clean diaper, washcloth, basin of water, soap, and powder.
5. Assist patient to lie on his or her back.
6. Explain the procedure to the patient before proceeding.
7. Remove the front portion of the diaper first and roll as close to the patient as possible, containing the waste inside the rolled diaper.
8. Thoroughly wash the skin of the lower abdomen, sides, and then the genitalia with soap and water.
9. Rinse well and dry.
10. Assist the patient to turn onto the side.
11. Using the same rolling pattern, remove the entire diaper. Thoroughly wash the skin of the buttocks and rectal area with soap and water.
12. Rinse well and dry.

13. Observe the skin for any signs of breakdown. Report breakdown areas to your supervisor.
14. Place powder around genitalia to absorb any remaining moisture.
15. Place the diaper behind the patient.
16. Assist the patient to roll onto his or her back.
17. Pull the diaper through the legs and up over the lower abdomen.
18. Secure the diaper using tape (disposable diapers) or safety pins, pointing downward (cloth diapers).
19. Replace clothing.
20. Assist patient to a comfortable location.
21. Wash washcloths and soiled cloth diaper. Place in a pail or isolated hamper.
22. Remove gloves.
23. Wash hands.
24. Document procedure.

## Nail Care

1. Do *not* cut the nails of any diabetic patient or patient with circulation problems.
2. Cut nails only with the approval of the nurse on your written care plan.
3. Wash hands.

4. Gather supplies (basin, soapy water, nail cutter, orange stick, washcloth, towel).
5. Explain procedure to patient.
6. Soak patient's hands and/or feet in a basin of warm, soapy water for about five minutes.
7. Wash patient's hands and/or feet and dry thoroughly.
8. Cut nails, leaving enough nail to allow white to show under the entire nail.
9. File any rough edges from nails.
10. Push cuticles back with the orange stick.
11. Assist patient to put on socks and shoes.
12. Return supplies to their location.
13. Wash hands.
14. Document procedure.

## Oral Hygiene/Denture Care

1. Ask patient for permission to clean dentures and assist with oral hygiene.
2. Wash hands.
3. Put on nonsterile gloves.
4. Ask patient to remove dentures.
5. Place dentures in a denture cup filled halfway with water.
6. Brush dentures with denture product and separate toothbrush.

7. Soak dentures in a denture cleanser as you continue with oral care.
8. Brush any remaining teeth with toothpaste and a toothbrush.
9. Clean upper and lower gums with a dampened cloth or tooth sponge product.
10. Ask patient to rinse with mouthwash.
11. Rinse dentures.
12. Give dentures back to patient to put in place.
13. Return supplies to their appropriate location.
14. Take gloves off.
15. Wash hands.
16. Document procedure.

## Application of Elastic Stockings

1. Remove and apply elastic stockings only if ordered to do so on the aide care plan.
2. Wash hands.
3. Remove elastic stockings.
4. Assess legs for discoloration, pain, and temperature extremes.
5. Report any problems to your supervisor.
6. Wash and thoroughly dry the legs.
7. Apply moisturizing lotion and allow to dry thoroughly.
8. Dust ankles with talcum powder to make application of elastic stockings easier.

9. Insert your hand into elastic stocking from the stocking top down to the open toe.
10. Stretch the foot section with your index and middle fingers of both hands.
11. Ease elastic stocking over patient's toes, stretching the stocking sideways as you move it up patient's foot.
12. Ask patient to push against your force as you ease the stocking up the leg.
13. Adjust the top of the elastic stocking one or two inches below patient's knee.
14. Assess the elastic stocking for wrinkles.
15. Smooth all wrinkles.
16. Wash hands.
17. Check patient's toes at least every four hours or as indicated by condition.
18. Launder elastic stockings with mild soap and lukewarm water as necessary. Do not put in a clothes dryer.
19. Document the removal and application of elastic stockings.

## Application of a Condom Catheter

1. Explain the procedure to the patient.
2. Wash hands.
3. Put on nonsterile gloves.

4. Wash penis and scrotum with soap and water. Rinse well. Dry.
5. Assess shaft of penis and scrotum for irritation, swelling, or excretions.
6. Roll condom catheter over the penis, leaving approximately one inch between the end of the penis and the catheter.
7. Assess for a snug but not tight fit.
8. Secure condom catheter with the tape supplied by the manufacturer. Follow the manufacturer's guidelines.
9. Connect the adapter to tubing/bag.
10. Remove gloves.
11. Wash hands.
12. Document procedure.

## Routine Catheter Care

1. Wash hands.
2. Put on nonsterile gloves.
3. Gather supplies, as needed (catheter bag, basin, antibacterial soap, washcloth, towel).
4. Explain procedure to patient.
5. Cleanse the catheter and area around its entrance into the body with warm water and soap.
6. Rinse well with water, and pat dry.

7. If your patient is an uncircumcised male, roll the foreskin back to clean underneath with soap and water, dry well, and replace foreskin to its natural position over the head of the penis.
8. Make sure that the catheter is secured with a leg strap in a position of comfort.
9. Return supplies to their appropriate location.
10. Remove gloves.
11. Wash hands.
12. Document procedure.

## Catheter Maintenance

The following are general guidelines for caring for a patient with an indwelling catheter:

1. Keep the bag below the level of the patient's bladder (pelvis) to foster good drainage.
2. Check the level of urine in the bag to make sure that urine is still flowing into it.
3. Position the catheter tube to stop it from being pulled out. You may use a piece of tape or a catheter strap.

4. Empty the contents of the bag every eight hours or with every visit (whichever is more often).
5. Call your supervisor in the following situations:
   - The catheter stops draining. (Before calling the supervisor, check to make sure that the tubing is not kinked.)
   - The patient complains of pain.
   - The urine is cloudy or foul smelling.
6. Clean any bags not in use as follows:
   - Put on nonsterile gloves.
   - Empty the urine into the commode.
   - Run warm/hot water through the bag.
   - Add two or three ounces of white vinegar to the water in the bag and let it sit for about 20 minutes to remove any residue (scum).
   - Rinse and dry.
   - Clean the end with alcohol prior to inserting it into the catheter at the time of the next change.
   - Remove gloves.
   - Wash hands.
7. Document procedure.

## Cleansing of Artificial Eye

1. Ask the patient to tell you his or her routine for artificial eye care.
2. Instruct patient and/or family/caregiver about the procedure.

3. Assist the patient to a semi-Fowler's position.
4. Gather supplies (nonsterile gloves, basin, wet washcloth, cotton balls, antibacterial soap, additional lighting, if needed).
5. Wash hands.
6. Put on nonsterile gloves.
7. Cover the bottom of small basin with a wet washcloth.
8. Cleanse eyelids with moistened cotton ball.
9. Push the upper eyelid upward with index finger.
10. Push the lower eyelid downward with thumb to break suction.
11. Cup other hand under eye socket to catch the artificial eye.
12. Clean the artificial eye with mild soap and water by rubbing between index finger and thumb.
13. Rinse the artificial eye in warm water.
14. Cleanse edge of eye socket from near the bridge of the nose outward with moistened cotton balls.
15. Reinsert eye by raising upper eyelid with index finger and thumb.
16. Slip artificial eye, with marked edge toward nose, up under eyelid.
17. Press lower eyelid down and allow the artificial eye to slide into socket.
18. Pull upper eyelid forward and down to cover eye and hold securely into place.

19. Wipe eyelids with moistened cotton ball, wiping toward nose to prevent dislodging.
20. Wipe nose.
21. Remove, clean, and return supplies to appropriate storage.
22. Remove gloves.
23. Wash hands.
24. Document procedure.

## Making an Occupied Bed

1. Wash hands.
2. Put on nonsterile gloves if bed is soiled or there is a chance of patient being incontinent.
3. Explain the procedure to the patient.
4. Gather supplies (linens, protective bed pads).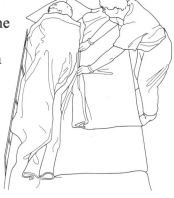
5. Raise the side rail on the far side of the bed.
6. Assist patient to turn toward you and lie as close to the side of the bed as possible.
7. Move to the opposite side of the bed and lower the side rail in front of you.

8. Untuck the dirty bottom sheet(s) and roll them toward the patient.
9. Gently tuck the sheets under the patient.
10. Open a clean sheet and lay it lengthwise on the uncovered portion of the mattress, aligning the bottom edge of the sheet with the edge of the mattress at the foot of the bed.
11. Tuck the excess sheet at the head of the bed under the mattress.
12. Fold back the upper corner to form a triangle, and tuck the excess under the mattress.
13. Tuck the side of the sheet under the mattress.
14. Roll the remainder of the sheet toward the center of the bed and gently tuck it under the rolled dirty sheet.
15. Place a protective pad under the patient's buttock, and again roll and tuck the excess under the patient.
16. Place the side rail on the opposite side of the bed into the upright position.
17. Assist the patient to roll over the tucked sheets toward you and onto his or her opposite side.
18. Move to the other side of the bed.
19. Lower the side rail in front of you.
20. Pull the dirty sheets through and place in a hamper.
21. Pull the clean sheets through, and tuck the excess sheet at the head of the bed under the mattress.

22. Fold back the upper corner to form a triangle, and tuck the excess under the mattress.
23. Pull the sheet tight and tuck under the mattress.
24. Assist the patient into a position of comfort.
25. Cover the patient with sheet and blankets, as appropriate.
26. Remove the patient's pillow and replace the pillow cover.
27. Position the pillow to a position of comfort.
28. Remove gloves.
29. Wash hands.
30. Document procedure.

## Making an Unoccupied Bed

1. Wash hands.
2. Put on nonsterile gloves, if linens are soiled.
3. Explain the need to change the linens to the patient.
4. Gather supplies (linens, protective bed pads).
5. Lower the side rails, if up.
6. Assist the patient to a chair.
7. Remove the dirty sheets and pillow cover and place them in the hamper.
8. Open a clean sheet and lay it over the uncovered mattress, aligning the bottom edge of the sheet with the edge of the mattress at the foot of the bed.

9. Tuck the excess sheet at the head of the bed under the mattress.
10. Fold back the upper corner to form a triangle, and tuck the excess under the mattress.
11. Tuck the side of the sheet under the mattress.
12. Move to the other side of the bed.
13. Tuck the excess sheet at the head of the bed under the mattress.
14. Fold back the upper corner to form a triangle, and tuck the excess under the mattress.
15. Pull the sheet tight and tuck under the mattress.
16. Open the clean top sheet over the newly covered mattress, leaving the excess at the bottom of the bed.
17. Tuck the excess under the mattress and fold back edges into triangles, tucking the excess under the mattress on both sides.
18. Fanfold the top sheet to the bottom of the bed.
19. Place a protective cover over the center portion of the mattress, if needed.
20. Replace the pillow cover.
21. Remove gloves, if worn.
22. Wash hands.
23. Document procedure.

## Shaving

1. Wash hands.
2. Check razor for condition:
   - sharp
   - clean
   - rust free
3. Position patient as follows:
   - If appropriate, place conscious patient in high Fowler or semi-Fowler position.
   - If appropriate, place unconscious patient with head elevated.
4. Adjust lighting in room to provide lighted area for shaving.
5. Straight or safety razor shave:
   - Fill wash basin with warm water (approximately 105°–110° Fahrenheit).
   - Check temperature with inner wrist.

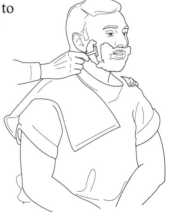

- Place towel around the shoulders, and tuck under patient's chin.
- Soak entire beard with warm, wet washcloth for approximately two minutes.
- Apply shaving cream or lathered soap to the beard.
- Gently pull the skin taut with one hand while shaving patient's beard with other hand.
- Begin with sideburns and work toward the chin.
- Use short, firm, downward strokes in the direction of hair growth.
- Rinse razor blade frequently.
- Apply additional warm water or shaving cream to patient's face if needed.
- Shave across the chin and up the neck and throat.
- Use short, gentle strokes for the neck and area around the nose and mouth.
- Change water.
- Rinse remaining shaving cream or lathered soap and hair from patient's face.
- Pat face dry.

6. Electric razor shave:
   - Plug in electric razor.
   - Apply preshave lotion.
   - Select setting of electric razor.
   - Shave each area of the face until it is smooth.

    • Use circular motion.

    • Press electric razor firmly against patient's skin.

7. Apply after-shave lotion or talcum powder, if desired.
8. Remove, clean, and store shaving equipment.
9. Place soiled linen in dirty laundry.
10. Wash hands.
11. Document procedure.

## Shampoo in Sink

1. Instruct patient about the procedure.
2. Wash hands.
3. Assist patient to the bathroom or kitchen sink area.
4. Start water, and set temperature to approximately 105°–110° Fahrenheit.
5. Check temperature of water on inner wrist.
6. Position patient in a comfortable position with head over sink.
7. Thoroughly wet hair and scalp with water.
8. Apply shampoo to patient's hair, and work it into a lather.
9. Rinse shampoo from hair.
10. Repeat steps 7–9.
11. Apply conditioner if desired, and rinse.
12. Towel dry and comb hair.

13. Remove, clean, and store equipment.
14. Wash hands
15. Document procedure.

**Shampoo in Bed**

1. Instruct patient or family/caregiver about the procedure.
2. Wash hands.
3. Position patient with head and shoulders close to edge of bed.
4. Place moisture-protection barrier to create a water trough, or use inflated shampoo tray.
5. Thoroughly wet patient's hair and scalp with water at approximately 105°–110° F.
6. Check water temperature with inner wrist.
7. Apply shampoo to hair, and work it into a lather.
8. Rinse shampoo from hair.
9. Repeat steps 6–8.
10. Apply conditioner if desired, and rinse.
11. Towel dry and comb hair.
12. Remove, clean, and store equipment.
13. Wash hands.
14. Document procedure.

**Positioning**

1. Position changes should be made at least every two hours.

2. Explain the procedure to the patient.
3. Wash hands.
4. Ask the patient his or her position preference.
5. Remove any pillows and bed covers to allow free movement.
6. Assist the patient with turning, as needed. If the patient asks to be allowed to turn independently, be patient and honor the request.
7. Patients should be positioned for comfort. The position should allow all joints to be in good alignment, which means:
   • The shoulders are back.
   • Pillows are used to support legs and arms.
   • Pillows are securely tucked to support the torso.
8. Make sure the patient is comfortable.
9. Cover the patient.
10. Wash hands.

## Range of Motion

1. Perform range of motion exercises only when approved to do so by the nurse on your aide care plan.

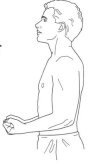
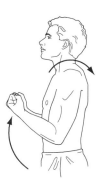

2. Generally, any bed-bound patient should have range of motion exercises to prevent contractures (in which muscles shorten and do not allow joints to move).
3. Wash hands.
4. Remove covers that would restrict the movement of the joint being exercised.
5. Ask the patient to do the exercise (active range of motion), or perform the exercise for the patient (passive range of motion).
6. Move each joint through its normal movements. If in doubt, move your joints to see how they move.
   • shoulders, hips, wrists, and ankles: rotate, move forward and backward, move side to side
   • knees and elbows: bend, extend straight
   • fingers: make a fist, extend outward, fan open and closed
   • toes: bend, extend outward
   • back (range of motion usually obtained through positioning): bends, extends straight
7. Repeat every movement 5 times at first, and gradually work up to 10 times.
8. Reposition patient for comfort when done.
9. Cover patient.
10. Wash hands.

## Log Rolling

Log rolling is used for patients with back problems or severe pain. When log rolling, the patient's back is not bent or twisted in any way. It keeps the back in alignment during position changes.

1. Explain the procedure to the patient.
2. Remove covers and pillow from under head.
3. Put side rail down.
4. Lean over patient with knees bent.
5. Place your lower arm firmly at the patient's hips and your other lower arm at the patient's shoulder level.
6. At the count of three, roll the patient toward you in one continuous motion.
7. Support the patient with pillows.

8. Make sure the patient is comfortable.
9. Cover the patient.
10. Wash hands.

## Transfer from Lying to Sitting on Side of Bed

1. Wash hands.
2. Explain the procedure to the patient.
3. Ask the patient to assist with the transfer.
4. Put the side rail down.
5. Align the patient straight in the bed.
6. Turn the patient on his or her side at the edge of the bed.
7. Unassisted:
   - Have the patient push down on the bed with his or her hands, which will elevate the upper torso.
   - At the same time the patient should push the lower extremities over the edge of the bed.
8. Assisted:
   - Place one hand under the patient's shoulder and the other at the patient's thigh.
   - At the count of three, assist the patient to pivot to a sitting position.
9. Wash hands.

## Backrub

1. Wash hands.
2. Gather supplies (lotion, talcum powder).
3. Provide for patient's privacy.

4. Assist patient to remove clothing on upper torso.
5. Ask patient to roll onto stomach.
6. Place lotion in hands and warm it by rubbing hands together.
7. Begin with long strokes at the base of the spine, as follows:
   • With hands side by side, rub up to the shoulders along the spinal column.
   • Separating hands, go around the shoulders.
   • Rub down the outsides of the back, and join hands at the base of the spine.
   • Repeat this movement at least four times.
8. Proceed to a spiral motion, as follows:
   • With hands side by side, rub up to the shoulders along the spinal column.
   • Separating hands, go around the shoulders.
   • Rub in short, circular patterns down the outsides of the back and join hands at the base of the spine.
   • Repeat this movement for at least three minutes.
9. End with at least four movements described above in step 7.
10. Assist the patient to dress.
11. Wash hands.

**Vital Signs**

All vital statistic measurements are to be documented within the clinical record.

1. Assess the patient's vital signs upon admission and then as indicated by the plan of care and patient condition.
2. Gather equipment (blood pressure cuff, stethoscope, thermometer).
3. Check the equipment for function and repair.

### Blood Pressure

1. Take the blood pressure in the same arm each time.
2. Place the blood pressure cuff on the upper arm approximately one inch above the antecubital fossa.
3. Palpate the patient's pulse in the inside bend of the elbow.
4. Place the diaphragm of the stethoscope over this pulse site.
5. Tighten the thumbscrew at the bulb of the blood pressure cuff.
6. Pump air into the cuff by pressing and releasing the bulb until the mercury rises to approximately 150–180 mm of pressure.
7. Slowly release the air from the cuff while listening closely. Record the number at the needle when the first sound (systolic) is heard and then the number when the last sound (diastolic) is heard.
8. Call your supervisor and/or the nurse when the top number is below 90 or over 180 or the bottom number is below 50 or over 100. These vital signs should be reported to the physician.

## Pulse Rate

Take the pulse in the location identified by the nurse on the aide care plan. Call your supervisor and/or the nurse if the pulse is below 60 or above 100.

*Apical Pulse.*
1. Warm the stethoscope diaphragm.
2. Place the diaphragm at the apex of the heart (on the anterior chest at the fifth intercostal space at the left mid-clavicular line).
3. Count the heart beats for one full minute, using a watch or clock with a second hand.
4. Note the rhythm. Is it regular and rhythmic or ir-regular? Report any irregularity.

*Radial Pulse.*
1. Place your index and middle fingers on the thumbside of the patient's wrist to locate the radial pulse.
2. Count the pulse rate for 15 seconds, using a watch or clock with a second hand.
3. Multiply your 15-second count by 4 to get the patient's radial pulse.

## Respiration

Evaluate the patient's breathing every time you check the pulse.

1. Assess the patient's respiration for frequency and rhythm over a one-minute time period. Normal respirations are of equal rhythm and a rate between 16 and 20 breaths per minute.
2. Call your supervisor and/or the nurse if the breathing rate is below 12 or greater than 24. These findings require physician notification.

### *Temperature*

The temperature is assessed by the most appropriate route. When glass thermometers are used, the mercury is shaken down to below 97 degrees Fahrenheit.

*Rectal Temperature.*
1. Assess temperature rectally for unconscious patients, irrational patients, patients with mouth disease, infants, children, and patients with recent nasal or oral surgery.
2. Always mark any thermometer used for rectal temperatures "for rectal temperatures only."
3. Cover thermometer with a plastic sheath.
4. Put on nonsterile gloves.
5. Apply water-soluble lubricant to the thermometer with a gloved hand.
6. Insert the thermometer gently into the rectum, as follows:
   • approximately 1½ inches for adults

- approximately ½ to 1 inch for children
- approximately ¼ to ½ inch for newborns and infants

7. Hold the thermometer in place throughout the procedure for newborn infants, children, and confused adults.

8. Remove glass thermometers after five minutes and electronic thermometers after they signal completion.

9. Read the temperature and document.

10. Remove the sheath, and cleanse the thermometer with alcohol.

11. Remove gloves.

12. Wash hands.

*Oral Temperature.*

1. Assess the temperature orally whenever the patient is cooperative and his or her condition does not contraindicate oral temperature assessment.

2. Use a glass oral thermometer or an electronic thermometer.

3. Cover the thermometer with a plastic sheath.

4. Place the thermometer gently under the tongue.

5. Remove the glass thermometer after three minutes and the electronic thermometer after it signals completion.

6. Read the temperature and document.

7. Remove the sheath, and cleanse the thermometer with alcohol.
8. Remove gloves and wash hands.

## Collecting Specimens

Home care aides are sometimes asked to assist with the collection of specimens that may not be available when the nurse or respiratory therapist is with the patient. The nurse or therapist should give you complete instructions when this is necessary. Some common specimen needs and collection steps follow:

### *Urine Specimens (Nonsterile)*

1. Explain the procedure to the patient.
2. Wash hands.
3. Gather equipment (gloves, clean specimen container).
4. Put on nonsterile gloves.
5. Cleanse the patient's perineal area with soap and water.
6. Instruct the patient to urinate into the specimen container.
7. Ask the patient to complete the flow into the toilet or bedpan.
8. Place the lid securely on the container.

9. Assist the patient with wiping and dressing.
10. If not done by the nurse, label the container with
    - patient's name
    - date
    - type of specimen
    - time of collection
    - physician name
11. Place the specimen in a plastic bag and then into a brown paper bag.
12. Remove gloves.
13. Wash hands.
14. Refrigerate the specimen.
15. Notify the nurse or your supervisor that the specimen is ready.
16. Document the procedure and the communication to the nurse or supervisor.

### Urine Testing with Reagent Strips

1. Explain the procedure to the patient.
2. Gather supplies (reagent strips, nonsterile gloves, specimen container).
3. Put on nonsterile gloves.
4. Ask patient to void approximately 30 cc's into the specimen container. Do not use the first A.M. voiding.
5. Remove reagent strip from container, taking caution not to touch the test strip area.

6. Immediately replace the cap securely.
7. Reference the label on the container for exact timing of test.
8. Dip the reagent strip into the newly collected specimen. While removing it, gently drag the strip against the side of the container to remove excess urine.
9. Begin counting the seconds immediately.
10. At the exact time noted on the container, compare the color of the reagent strip to the container color descriptions.
11. Remove gloves.
12. Wash hands.
13. Document the time, procedure, and result of the test.
14. Communicate the results to the nurse and/or your supervisor, as requested.

### Stool Specimen

1. Explain the procedure to the patient.
2. Wash hands.
3. Gather equipment (gloves, clean specimen container, tongue blade).
4. Put on nonsterile gloves.
5. Instruct the patient to use a bedpan. If a bedpan is not available, have the patient use the toilet.
6. Instruct the patient:
   • not to urinate with the bowel movement

- not to flush the toilet after having a bowel movement
- to place the soiled toilet tissue on a piece of paper towel

7. When the patient is finished, obtain a small piece of the stool and place it in the container.
8. Discard the toilet tissue.
9. Flush the waste products down the toilet.
10. Place the lid securely on the container.
11. If not done by the nurse, label the container with
    - patient's name
    - date
    - type of specimen
    - time of collection
    - physician name
12. Place the specimen in a plastic bag and then into a brown paper bag.
13. Remove gloves.
14. Wash hands.
15. Refrigerate the specimen.
16. Notify the nurse or your supervisor that the specimen is ready.
17. Document the procedure and the communication to the nurse or supervisor.

# Bibliography

Ahmann, E. 1996. *Home care for the high-risk infant: A family-centered approach.* 2d ed. Gaithersburg, MD: Aspen Publishers, Inc.

American Association of Retired Persons. 1993. *A profile of older Americans.* Washington, DC: Author.

American National Red Cross. 1972. *First aid.* 4th ed. Garden City, NY: Doubleday and Co.

Bassett, L.C., and N. Metzger. 1986. *Achieving excellence.* Gaithersburg, MD: Aspen Publishers, Inc.

Belasco, J. 1991. *Teaching the elephant to dance, A manager's guide to empowering change.* New York: Crown Publishers.

Bennett, G. 1994. *The McGraw Hill 36 hour management course.* New York: McGraw Hill Publishers.

Berne, E. 1964. *Games people play.* New York: Ballantine Books.

Branch, M.F., and P.P. Paxton. 1976. *Providing safe nursing care for ethnic people of color.* New York: Appleton-Century-Crofts.

Canfield, S. June 1995. Pre-employment inquiries. St. Joseph Hospital education session. Lancaster, PA.

Development Dimensions International. 1987. *Interaction management.* Pittsburgh, PA: DDI Press.

Ellis, M. 1997. Preventing back injury—Inservice. *The Home Health Aide Educator* 1, no. 2: 1–6. York, PA: ADVANTAGE Health Care Management Resources Press.

Getting along with the boss. 1998. *The Home Health Aide Educator* 1, no. 3: 4. York, PA: Advantage Health Care Management Resources Press.

Gingerich, B.S., and D.A. Ondeck. 1995. *Clinical Pathways for the Multidisciplinary Home Care Team.* Supplement 5, November 1997. Gaithersburg, MD: Aspen Publishers, Inc.

Gingerich, B.S., and D.A. Ondeck. 1995. *Home health care job descriptions and performance appraisals.* York, PA: ADVANTAGE Health Care Management Resources Press.

Gingerich, B.S., and D.A. Ondeck. 1996. *Infection control program for the home care organization.* 2d ed. York, PA: ADVANTAGE Health Care Management Resources Press.

Gingerich, B.S., and D.A. Ondeck. 1996. *Safety manual for the home care organization.* 2d ed. York, PA: ADVANTAGE Health Care Management Resources Press.

Green, K. 1996. *Home health aide training manual.* Gaithersburg, MD: Aspen Publishers, Inc.

Harris, D.K. 1990. *Sociology of aging.* 2d ed. New York: Harper and Row.

Henry, O., and G. Henry. 1997. Developing a workplace violence program in the home health care setting. *Home Health Care Management and Practice* 9, no. 4: 14–21.

*The Home Health Aide Educator.* 1997–1998. ADVANTAGE Health Care Management Resources Press.

Katzenbach, J.R., and D.K. Smith. 1993. *The wisdom of teams.* New York: Harper Business Publisher.

Keirsey, D., and M. Bates. 1984. *Please understand me character & temperament types.* 4th ed. Del Mar, CA: Prometheus Nemesis Book Company.

Kimmel, D.C. 1974. *Adulthood and aging.* New York: Wiley, pp. 369–376.

Kubler-Ross, E. 1997. *On death and dying.* London: Collier Books.

La Ferriere, R., et al. 1996. Evaluating work satisfaction of paraprofessionals in home health care. *Home Health Care Management and Practice* 8, no. 2: 21–28.

Levinson, D.J. 1978. *The seasons of a man's life.* New York: Ballantine Books.

McCallister, L. 1992. *"I wish I'd said that!" How to talk your way out of trouble and into success.* New York: John Wiley & Sons, Inc.

McMurtry, A. 1997. Rub-a-dub-dub, An aide in the tub. *The Home Health Aide Educator* 1, no. 1: 3. York, PA: ADVANTAGE Health Care Management Resources Press.

*Medicare Home Health Agency Manual.* 1995. HCFA-Pub. 11. Washington, D.C.

*Myers-Briggs Type Indicator.* 1991. Palo Alto, CA: Consulting Psychologists Press, Inc.

National Association for Home Care. 1997. *1997 National homecare & hospice directory.* 9th ed. Washington, D.C.

Para, P. 1998. Worker security and violence in the workplace. Paper presented at the National Association for Home Care Region X Conference. Portland, OR.

*Reader's Digest great encyclopedic dictionary.* 1975. Pleasantville, NY: Funk and Wagnalls Publishing Company, Inc.

Schaffer, R. July 1993. Interviewing. Educational Sessions at the Joint Commission on Accreditation of Healthcare Organizations. Oakbrook Terrace, IL.

Schaffer, R. July 1994. Communications and Group Dynamics. Educational Sessions at the Joint Commission on Accreditation of Healthcare Organizations. Oakbrook Terrace, IL.

Schmidt, K. 1996. Professional development of home health care aides: The key to retention. *Home Health Care Management and Practice* 8, no. 3: 7–13.

Scholtes, P. et al. 1991. *The team handbook—How to use teams to improve quality.* Madison, WI: Joiner Associates.

Spector, R.E., and I.K. Zola. 1979. *Cultural diversity in health and illness.* New York: Appleton-Century-Crofts.

Stevenson, J.S. 1977. *Issues and crises during middlescence.* New York: Appleton-Century-Crofts, pp. 18, 25.

Thobaben, M., and W. Woodward. 1996. Workplace security for home health care employees. *Home Health Care Management and Practice* 8, no. 6: 58–65.

Wernig, J., and S. Sorrentino. 1989. *The homemaker-home health aide.* St. Louis, MO: CV Mosby.

Willborn, E.H. 1988. *Manual for the homemaker/home health aide.* Philadelphia: J.B. Lippincott Co.

Zucker, E. 1996. *Being a homemaker/home health aide.* 4th ed. Upper Saddle River, NJ: Brady Prentice Hall.

# Index